NURSING DRUG GUIDE

Essential Pharmacology, Drug Dosages, and Safe Medication Administration for Effective and Confident Nursing Practice — Master Medication Management and Prevent Critical Errors

VICTORIA HART

© 2025 Nursing Drug guide All rights reserved. This material is intended solely for

educational purposes related to 'Nursing Drug guide'.' The book is offered 'as is,' with no
guarantees of any kind, whether stated or implied. The publisher assumes no liability for any
harm or loss resulting from the application or misapplication of the information presented in
this book. All trademarks and brand names mentioned herein are the property of their
respective owners and are used only for identification purposes. Any unauthorized
reproduction, distribution, or transmission of this book, in whole or in part, is strictly forbidden.

SCAN THE QR CODE TO DOWNLOAD

YOUR BONUS

TABLE OF CONTENTS

1. INTRODUCTION 5
    1.1 Purpose of this Guide Purpose of This Guide.. 5
    1.2 How to Use this Guide 8
    1.3 Core Principles of Pharmacology... 11
  2. SAFE MEDICATION ADMINISTRATION... 15
    2.1 Dosage Calculations and Essential Conversions................................. 19
    2.3 The "Rights" of Medication Administration....................................... 23
    2.4 Preventing Medication Errors 27
    2.5 Monitoring for Adverse Reactions... 30
  3. HIGH-ALERT DRUGS & SAFETY WARNINGS 35
    3.1 High-Risk Medications (Anticoagulants, Insulin, Opioids) 35
    3.2 Black Box Warnings: What Nurses Need to Know............................. 38
    3.3 Risk Reduction Strategies 41
  4. DRUG CLASSIFICATIONS: NURSING ESSENTIALS 45
    4.1 – Antibiotics and Antimicrobials (Extended List with Dosages)........ 45
    4.2 – Cardiovascular Drugs (Extended, 70+ Drugs)................................. 48
    4.3 – Analgesics and Anti-Inflammatory Drugs (Extended List) 59
    4.4 – Central Nervous System Medications (Extended List)............**Error! Bookmark not defined.**
    4.5 – Endocrine and Metabolic Medications (Extended List).................. 73
    4.6 – Gastrointestinal Medications (Extended List) 79
    4.7 – Respiratory Medications (Extended List) 84
    4.8 – Immune System Medications (Extended List)................................ 90
    4.9 – Renal and Urinary Medications (Extended List) 95
    4.10 – Women's and Men's Health Medications (Extended List).......... 100
  5. ADVERSE EFFECTS & DRUG INTERACTIONS... 106
    5.1 Recognizing Adverse Drug Reactions (ADRs) 106
    5.2 Reporting & Managing Reactions 109
    5.3 Common Drug-Drug & Drug-Food Interactions 112
  6. IV DRUG ADMINISTRATION GUIDELINES 117
    6.1 IV Compatibility & Mixing Chart 117
    6.2 IV Push vs Drip: Rate & Safety 121
    6.3 Preventing IV Site Complications 125
  7. HERBAL, OTC & ALTERNATIVE MEDICATIONS 130

- *7.1 Common Supplements & Patient Use* 130
- *7.2 Key Interactions with Prescription Drugs* 134
- *7.3 Counseling Patients on Safe Use* 137
8. SPECIAL POPULATIONS & CLINICAL SCENARIOS 140
   - *8.1 Emergency & Critical Care Drugs* 140
   - *8.2 Pregnancy & Lactation Considerations* 144
   - *8.3 Pediatric Dosing & Safety* 149
   - *8.4 Geriatric Medication Management* 153
9. CLINICAL NURSING PRACTICE 157
   - *9.1 The 10 Golden Rules of Drug Safety* 157
   - *9.2 Teaching Patients About Their Medications* 160
   - *9.3 Proper Medication Documentation* 164
10. DOSAGE & IV CALCULATIONS CHEAT SHEET 168
    - *10.1 Weight-Based & Pediatric Dosing* 168
    - *10.2 IV Flow Rate Calculations* 172
    - *10.3 Common Conversion Charts* 176
11. CLINICAL CASE STUDIES 180
    - *11.1 Real-World Medication Errors* 180
    - *11.2 Managing Reactions in Practice* 185
    - *11.3 Medication Safety in Action* 189
12. APPENDICES & RESOURCES 194
    - *12.1 Common Abbreviations in Pharmacology* 194
    - *12.2 Glossary of Key Terms* 201
    - *12.3 Conversion Charts & Units* 205
    - *12.4 Most Commonly Prescribed Drugs (U.S. 2025)* 210

1. INTRODUCTION

1.1 PURPOSE OF THIS GUIDE
PURPOSE OF THIS GUIDE

The NURSING DRUG GUIDE 2025–2026 has been developed with one clear purpose: **to empower nurses with accurate, evidence-based, and clinically useful drug information** that supports safe and effective medication administration across all care settings. In today's fast-paced and high-acuity healthcare environments, nurses must make swift, informed decisions—often under pressure. This guide serves as a dependable point-of-care resource that helps ensure those decisions are grounded in sound pharmacological knowledge.

Unlike traditional pharmacology textbooks, which are often dense and overly theoretical, this guide is designed to be **practical, portable, and nursing-focused**. Every section reflects the way nurses think, act, and care. From bedside administration to discharge teaching, from emergency interventions to chronic disease management, this guide supports nurses in their **critical role as medication safety advocates**.

Specifically, the guide aims to:

- **Promote medication safety** by providing updated information on drug dosages, side effects, interactions, black box warnings, and contraindications.
- **Support clinical decision-making** through concise summaries, comparison charts, and nursing considerations specific to each drug.
- **Bridge the knowledge-practice gap** by translating pharmacological theory into practical nursing applications at the bedside.
- **Assist in patient education** by offering clear, patient-friendly explanations of medication actions, expectations, and side effects.
- **Serve as a study aid** for nursing students preparing for exams, including the NCLEX, and as a reference for licensed nurses updating their practice.

In every page, this guide reflects the **nursing perspective**—acknowledging the unique responsibilities nurses carry when it comes to drug administration. Nurses are not just medication dispensers; they are **vigilant observers, educators, assessors, and advocates**. Whether you're double-checking a high-alert medication, calculating a pediatric dose, or teaching a patient about their new prescription, this book is your trusted companion.

Ultimately, the purpose of this guide is simple but essential:
To make medication knowledge accessible, actionable, and nurse-centered—because patient safety depends on it.

Purpose of This Guide

The Nursing Drug Guide 2025–2026 has been developed with one clear purpose: to empower nurses with accurate, evidence-based, and clinically useful drug information that supports safe and effective medication administration across all care settings. In today's fast-paced and high-acuity healthcare environments, nurses must make swift, informed decisions—often under pressure. This guide serves as a dependable point-of-care resource that helps ensure those decisions are grounded in sound pharmacological knowledge.

Unlike traditional pharmacology textbooks, which are often dense and overly theoretical, this guide is designed to be practical, portable, and nursing-focused. Every section reflects the way nurses think, act, and care. From bedside administration to discharge teaching, from emergency interventions to chronic disease management, this guide supports nurses in their critical role as medication safety advocates.

Specifically, the guide aims to:

Promote medication safety by providing updated information on drug dosages, side effects, interactions, black box warnings, and contraindications.

Support clinical decision-making through concise summaries, comparison charts, and nursing considerations specific to each drug.

Bridge the knowledge-practice gap by translating pharmacological theory into practical nursing applications at the bedside.

Assist in patient education by offering clear, patient-friendly explanations of medication actions, expectations, and side effects.

Serve as a study aid for nursing students preparing for exams, including the NCLEX, and as a reference for licensed nurses updating their practice.

In every page, this guide reflects the nursing perspective—acknowledging the unique responsibilities nurses carry when it comes to drug administration. Nurses are not just medication dispensers; they are vigilant observers, educators, assessors, and advocates. Whether you're double-checking a high-alert medication, calculating a pediatric dose, or teaching a patient about their new prescription, this book is your trusted companion.

Ultimately, the purpose of this guide is simple but essential:

To make medication knowledge accessible, actionable, and nurse-centered—because patient safety depends on it.

1.2 HOW TO USE THIS GUIDE

The NURSING DRUG GUIDE 2025–2026 is designed for **practical, point-of-care use**—whether you're at the bedside, preparing for a clinical shift, studying for exams, or reviewing protocols with your interdisciplinary team. It serves both as a **reference tool** and a **learning aid**, tailored to fit the fast-paced decision-making process nurses face every day.

To get the most out of this guide, here's how to navigate and apply it effectively:

UNDERSTAND THE STRUCTURE

Each drug entry or class-specific section follows a consistent format to promote quick reference and comprehension. This format includes:

- **Generic and Brand Names**: Both are listed to avoid confusion between trade names and active ingredients.
- **Drug Class**: Includes both PHARMACOLOGIC (mechanism-based) and THERAPEUTIC (use-based) classifications.
- **Indications**: Conditions and diseases the drug is commonly prescribed to treat.

- **Dosage & Administration**: Standard dosing ranges, routes (oral, IV, IM, etc.), and frequency—including pediatric, geriatric, and renal-adjusted doses when applicable.
- **Side Effects**: Categorized into COMMON and SERIOUS/ADVERSE effects to help prioritize monitoring.
- **Contraindications & Precautions**: Conditions or factors that increase the risk of harm.
- **Nursing Considerations**: Key assessments, labs to monitor, administration tips, and safety checks.
- **Patient Teaching**: What to educate the patient about—such as what to expect, when to report symptoms, or how to store/administer the drug properly.
- **Black Box Warnings**: These are prominently flagged with bold alerts for quick visibility.

USE TABS AND CATEGORIES

The guide is divided into logical sections:

- **Chapters 1–3** cover the foundations of pharmacology and safety.
- **Chapter 4** (reserved) will include comprehensive drug classifications and individual drug monographs.
- **Chapters 5–6** focus on side effects and interactions.
- **Chapters 7–9** provide advanced nursing guidance, IV compatibility, and herbal considerations.
- **Chapters 10–12** offer case studies, resources, and glossary terms.

You can use the **table of contents** to jump to a specific drug class or clinical topic, or use the **search function** (if using a digital version) to locate specific drugs or terms instantly.

AT THE BEDSIDE

Keep this guide accessible during medication passes, documentation, and assessments. It helps ensure:

- **Correct dosage confirmation**
- **Quick reminders for adverse reactions**
- **Fast patient education talking points**
- **Nursing interventions** specific to the medication

WHILE STUDYING OR PREPPING

Whether you're preparing for the NCLEX, a nursing school exam, or continuing education, use this guide to:

- Reinforce pharmacologic concepts
- Test yourself on drug actions, dosages, and side effects
- Practice identifying nursing interventions in sample scenarios

DURING PATIENT EDUCATION

Use the "Patient Teaching" points to:

- Clarify the purpose and effect of medications
- Explain proper timing and administration
- Highlight symptoms that require reporting
- Discuss potential drug interactions or lifestyle adjustments

ICONS, ALERTS, AND FORMATTING

Look out for:

- **Bold warnings** for life-threatening side effects

- **Icons** or labels for high-alert medications
- **Special notations** for pediatric, geriatric, or renal adjustments
- **Checklists** for IV preparation and compatibility

1.3 CORE PRINCIPLES OF PHARMACOLOGY

Pharmacology is the scientific foundation of medication administration and drug therapy. For nurses, understanding core pharmacological principles is essential not only for administering medications safely but also for anticipating drug effects, preventing harm, and educating patients effectively. These core principles can be divided into two major categories: **pharmacokinetics** and **pharmacodynamics**—each of which plays a vital role in how drugs behave in the body.

Pharmacokinetics: What the Body Does to the Drug

Pharmacokinetics describes the journey of a drug through the body, following four major processes:

1. **Absorption**
    - The process by which a drug enters the bloodstream from its site of administration (e.g., GI tract, skin, muscle, vein).
    - Influenced by factors such as route of administration, blood flow, pH, and drug formulation.
2. **Distribution**
    - The transport of the drug to tissues and organs after it enters circulation.
    - Depends on protein binding, blood-brain barrier permeability, and lipid solubility.
3. **Metabolism (Biotransformation)**

- The chemical alteration of the drug, primarily in the liver (via the cytochrome P450 enzyme system).
- Converts the drug into active or inactive forms and prepares it for excretion.

4. **Excretion**
   - The removal of drugs from the body, primarily through the kidneys (urine), but also via bile, sweat, saliva, or breast milk.
   - Impaired renal function can lead to drug accumulation and toxicity.

These processes affect the **onset, intensity,** and **duration** of a drug's action.

Pharmacodynamics: What the Drug Does to the Body

Pharmacodynamics refers to the biochemical and physiological effects of drugs and their mechanisms of action.

- **Mechanism of Action (MOA):** How a drug produces its effect, typically by binding to receptors, inhibiting enzymes, or interacting with ion channels or transporters.
- **Drug-Receptor Interactions:** Most drugs exert their effects by mimicking or blocking the actions of the body's own chemical messengers (e.g., neurotransmitters, hormones).
- **Dose-Response Relationship:** The correlation between the drug dose and the magnitude of the effect. Understanding this helps determine the minimum effective dose and the maximum safe dose.
- **Therapeutic Index (TI):** The ratio between a drug's effective dose and its toxic dose. A narrow TI requires careful monitoring (e.g., warfarin, digoxin).
- **Potency vs. Efficacy:** Potency refers to how much drug is needed for effect, while efficacy is the drug's ability to produce a desired result.

Half-Life and Steady State

- **Half-Life (t½):** The time it takes for the plasma concentration of a drug to decrease by 50%. This determines dosing frequency.
- **Steady State:** Achieved when the rate of drug administration equals the rate of elimination—usually after 4–5 half-lives.

Bioavailability and First-Pass Effect

- **Bioavailability:** The fraction of the administered dose that reaches systemic circulation. IV drugs have 100% bioavailability; oral drugs usually have less.
- **First-Pass Effect:** Oral drugs may be metabolized in the liver before reaching systemic circulation, reducing their active concentration.

Factors That Influence Drug Action in Patients

- **Age:** Neonates and elderly patients may have altered metabolism or excretion.
- **Body weight and composition**
- **Genetics and enzyme function**
- **Renal and hepatic function**
- **Comorbidities and polypharmacy**
- **Tolerance, dependence, or resistance**

Nursing Application of Pharmacological Principles

Understanding pharmacology helps nurses:

- Choose correct timing and route of administration

- Monitor for adverse effects and therapeutic response
- Recognize signs of toxicity or drug ineffectiveness
- Anticipate drug interactions
- Educate patients on safe medication use

Pharmacology is not just about memorizing drugs—it's about applying knowledge critically to protect patients, personalize care, and improve outcomes.

2. SAFE MEDICATION ADMINISTRATION

2.1 ROUTES OF ADMINISTRATION (ORAL, IV, IM, SUBQ, ETC.)

The **route of administration** refers to the path by which a drug is taken into the body. The choice of route affects the **speed of absorption**, **bioavailability**, **onset of action**, and **potential for adverse effects**. Nurses must be familiar with each route to ensure **safe and effective medication administration**.

Below is an overview of the most common routes, their characteristics, and nursing implications:

ORAL (PO – PER OS)

- **Description:** Most common route; medication is swallowed and absorbed via the gastrointestinal (GI) tract.
- **Advantages:** Convenient, cost-effective, non-invasive.
- **Disadvantages:** Slower onset; affected by food, GI motility, and first-pass metabolism.
- **Nursing Considerations:**
    - Assess swallowing ability.
    - Administer with food if indicated or on an empty stomach if required.
    - Avoid crushing extended-release or enteric-coated tablets.

SUBLINGUAL (SL) AND BUCCAL

- **Description:** Medication is placed under the tongue (sublingual) or between the gum and cheek (buccal) for direct absorption into systemic circulation.
- **Advantages:** Rapid absorption; bypasses first-pass metabolism.
- **Disadvantages:** Limited to certain drugs; must remain in place until dissolved.
- **Nursing Considerations:**
    - Do not allow the patient to chew or swallow.
    - Avoid eating or drinking until fully absorbed.

INTRAVENOUS (IV)

- **Description:** Direct injection or infusion into the bloodstream.
- **Advantages:** Immediate onset; 100% bioavailability; precise control of dosage.
- **Disadvantages:** Invasive; risk of infection, phlebitis, infiltration.
- **Nursing Considerations:**
    - Verify IV site patency before administration.
    - Monitor for extravasation or allergic reactions.
    - Follow infusion protocols and rate guidelines.

INTRAMUSCULAR (IM)

- **Description:** Injection into muscle tissue (e.g., deltoid, vastus lateralis).
- **Advantages:** Faster absorption than subQ; suitable for depot formulations.
- **Disadvantages:** Can be painful; risk of nerve or vascular injury.
- **Nursing Considerations:**
    - Use appropriate needle length and site.
    - Rotate sites to prevent tissue damage.
    - Aspirate per facility policy before injecting.

SUBCUTANEOUS (SUBQ)

- **Description:** Injection into the fatty tissue beneath the skin (e.g., abdomen, thigh).
- **Advantages:** Slower, sustained absorption; ideal for insulin, heparin.
- **Disadvantages:** Limited volume capacity; potential site irritation.
- **Nursing Considerations:**
    - Use small gauge needles.
    - Do not massage after injection (especially for anticoagulants).
    - Rotate sites for long-term therapies.

TOPICAL AND TRANSDERMAL

- **Description:** Applied to skin or mucous membranes for local or systemic effects.
- **Advantages:** Non-invasive; sustained release possible (e.g., patches).
- **Disadvantages:** Skin irritation; variable absorption.
- **Nursing Considerations:**
    - Wear gloves when applying/removing.
    - Clean and dry skin before application.
    - Rotate transdermal patch sites; avoid heat over patch.

INHALATION

- **Description:** Drug is inhaled into the lungs via metered-dose inhalers (MDIs), dry powder inhalers (DPIs), or nebulizers.
- **Advantages:** Rapid absorption through alveoli; local effect for respiratory diseases.
- **Disadvantages:** Requires proper technique; coordination may be difficult.

- **Nursing Considerations:**
    - Educate on correct inhaler use.
    - Use spacers if needed.
    - Rinse mouth after corticosteroid inhalers.

RECTAL AND VAGINAL

- **Description:** Suppositories or creams inserted into the rectum or vagina.
- **Advantages:** Useful when oral route is not possible; local and systemic effects.
- **Disadvantages:** Inconvenient; absorption may be irregular.
- **Nursing Considerations:**
    - Maintain privacy and dignity.
    - Use gloves and lubrication.
    - Instruct patient to remain lying down after insertion.

OTHER ROUTES (ADVANCED/OCCASIONAL USE)

- **Intradermal (ID):** Allergy testing, tuberculosis screening.
- **Intraosseous (IO):** Emergency access to circulation through bone.
- **Intrathecal/Epidural:** Direct administration into spinal fluid for anesthesia or pain control.
- **Ophthalmic/Otic/Nasal:** Local administration to eye, ear, or nasal mucosa.

CHOOSING THE RIGHT ROUTE: KEY FACTORS

- Drug formulation and absorption profile

- Patient age, consciousness, and cooperation
- Condition being treated (local vs systemic)
- Need for rapid onset
- Risk of infection or complications

Proper knowledge of each route ensures **therapeutic effectiveness** and **minimizes risk**. Nurses play a key role in selecting, administering, and evaluating medications via the most appropriate route for each individual patient.

2.1 DOSAGE CALCULATIONS AND ESSENTIAL CONVERSIONS

Accurate dosage calculation is a critical nursing skill that directly impacts patient safety. Administering the wrong dose—even by a small margin—can lead to serious consequences, especially in vulnerable populations like children, older adults, or patients with renal or hepatic impairment.

This section provides a clear and concise guide to dosage calculations, essential conversions, and practical nursing applications.

CORE PRINCIPLES OF DOSAGE CALCULATION

To safely administer medication, nurses must be able to:

1. **Interpret medication orders accurately**
2. **Perform correct mathematical conversions**

3. Calculate doses based on weight or body surface area when indicated
4. Double-check high-risk medications or pediatric doses
5. Understand the medication's concentration, strength, and unit of measure

COMMON FORMULAS FOR DOSAGE CALCULATION

1. BASIC FORMULA (DESIRED OVER HAVE)

$$\text{Dose} = \frac{D}{H} \times Q$$

- **D** = Desired dose (what is ordered)
- **H** = Have (what is on hand)
- **Q** = Quantity (volume/tablets on hand)

Example:
Order: 500 mg
Available: 250 mg tablets

$$\frac{500}{250} \times 1 = 2\ \text{tablets}$$

2. WEIGHT-BASED DOSING

$$\text{Dose} = \text{mg/kg/day or mg/kg/dose} \times \text{weight in kg}$$

Example:
Order: 5 mg/kg/day for a child weighing 20 kg

$$5 \times 20 = 100\ \text{mg/day}$$

3. IV FLOW RATE (ML/HR)

$$\text{Rate} = \frac{\text{Volume (mL)}}{\text{Time (hr)}}$$

Example:
1000 mL over 8 hours

$$\frac{1000}{8} = 125 \text{ mL/hr}$$

4. DRIP RATE (GTT/MIN) FOR GRAVITY IVS

$$\text{gtt/min} = \frac{\text{Volume (mL)} \times \text{Drop Factor (gtt/mL)}}{\text{Time (min)}}$$

Example:
500 mL over 4 hours with a drop factor of 15 gtt/mL

$$\frac{500 \times 15}{240} = 31.25 \approx 31 \text{ gtt/min}$$

5. BODY SURFACE AREA (BSA) DOSING

$$\text{Dose} = \text{mg/m}^2 \times \text{BSA (m}^2\text{)}$$

BSA is commonly used in chemotherapy and pediatric medications.

ESSENTIAL UNIT CONVERSIONS

Metric Conversion	Approximate Equivalence
1 kg = 1000 g	1 g = 1000 mg
1 mg = 1000 mcg	1 L = 1000 mL
1 tsp = 5 mL	1 tbsp = 15 mL
1 oz = 30 mL	1 cup = 240 mL
1 inch = 2.54 cm	1 lb = 2.2 kg

1 mL = 1 cc (commonly used interchangeably in syringes)

PEDIATRIC DOSAGE CONSIDERATIONS

- Always **double-check** pediatric doses.
- Use **body weight in kilograms**—never in pounds.
- Double-verify **maximum daily doses**.
- Use **syringes with small increments** for liquid meds.
- Most errors occur from **misreading decimals**—extra zeros or lack of leading zeros can be fatal.

NURSING BEST PRACTICES

- Use a **calculator or dosing software** to reduce risk.
- Read labels **carefully**—some medications come in multiple strengths.
- Never guess or approximate doses—**ask if unsure**.
- Always **document** your calculation and administration promptly.
- For **high-risk medications** (e.g., heparin, insulin, opioids), perform **independent double-checks**.

RED FLAGS TO WATCH FOR

- Confusion between **mg and mcg**
- Misinterpretation of **IV concentrations**
- Decimal point misplacement (e.g., 1.0 mg vs 10 mg)
- Incorrect unit conversion between **mL and tsp**
- Dosing based on **actual vs ideal body weight** in specific populations (e.g., obesity)

2.3 THE "RIGHTS" OF MEDICATION ADMINISTRATION

The foundation of safe and accurate medication administration in nursing practice is built upon the established **"Rights" of Medication Administration**. Originally introduced as the "Five Rights," this framework has evolved to include a broader range of responsibilities, now encompassing ten or more rights recognized in modern clinical practice.

These rights serve as a structured guideline to reduce medication errors, enhance patient safety, and ensure accountability across all care settings. Every nurse should apply these principles consistently as part of standard clinical workflow.

1. RIGHT PATIENT

- Verify the patient's identity using two approved identifiers (e.g., full name and date of birth).
- Cross-check the identification band with the medication administration record (MAR).
- Exercise additional caution in non-verbal, unconscious, pediatric, or cognitively impaired patients.

2. RIGHT MEDICATION

- Confirm the exact name, formulation, and strength of the medication.
- Be vigilant with look-alike and sound-alike (LASA) medications.
- Always compare the medication label with the original order and the MAR before administration.

3. RIGHT DOSE

- Ensure the dose ordered matches the dose prepared, adjusting for patient-specific factors like weight or renal function.
- Perform necessary dosage calculations and verify with a second nurse if required.
- Take special care with high-risk medications such as insulin, heparin, and chemotherapy agents.

4. RIGHT ROUTE

- Confirm the ordered route of administration (oral, intravenous, intramuscular, subcutaneous, etc.).
- Assess patient factors that may contraindicate a specific route, such as dysphagia or vascular access limitations.
- Understand the implications of different routes on drug absorption and onset of action.

5. RIGHT TIME

- Administer medications at the time specified in the MAR or as clinically indicated.
- Clarify timing for time-critical medications such as antibiotics, insulin, or anticoagulants.
- Understand timing considerations related to meals, sleep cycles, or other treatments.

6. RIGHT DOCUMENTATION

- Accurately document all administered medications immediately after giving them.
- Include the time, route, dosage, and any relevant observations or patient responses.
- Record omitted or refused medications and provide appropriate follow-up.

7. RIGHT REASON

- Understand the clinical rationale for each medication.

- Verify that the prescribed drug is appropriate for the patient's diagnosis, condition, and current treatment plan.
- Be prepared to withhold a medication if it is no longer indicated and notify the prescriber.

8. RIGHT RESPONSE

- Monitor the patient's therapeutic and adverse responses after administration.
- Evaluate for effectiveness, especially with PRN medications.
- Report unexpected effects promptly and modify care as needed.

9. RIGHT EDUCATION

- Provide patients with clear, accurate information about the purpose of the medication, how it works, and what side effects to expect.
- Instruct on proper use for take-home medications, including storage and administration.
- Encourage patient questions and verify understanding to support adherence.

10. RIGHT TO REFUSE

- Recognize the patient's right to refuse any medication.
- Explore the reason for refusal with empathy and provide information as appropriate.
- Document the refusal and notify the healthcare provider when necessary.

CONCLUSION

The "Rights" of Medication Administration are more than a checklist—they represent a comprehensive, ethical, and clinical standard for medication safety. When applied consistently, they enhance patient care, reduce errors, and reinforce the nurse's role as a critical thinker and patient advocate. These principles should be internalized as part of daily nursing practice, ensuring that medication administration is always carried out with precision, professionalism, and care.

2.4 PREVENTING MEDICATION ERRORS

Medication errors are among the most common and preventable causes of harm in healthcare. They can occur at any stage of the medication process: prescribing, transcribing, dispensing, administering, or monitoring. Nurses play a vital role in identifying and preventing these errors, particularly at the point of administration.

This section outlines the most common types of medication errors, contributing factors, and evidence-based strategies for prevention in clinical nursing practice.

COMMON TYPES OF MEDICATION ERRORS

- **Wrong drug:** Administering a medication not ordered for the patient.
- **Wrong dose:** Giving too much, too little, or an incorrect concentration.
- **Wrong route:** Administering by the wrong method (e.g., IV instead of oral).
- **Wrong time:** Giving the medication too early, too late, or omitting a scheduled dose.

- **Wrong patient:** Failing to confirm identity properly.
- **Omission:** Failing to administer a necessary medication.
- **Unauthorized drug:** Administering a medication without a valid order.
- **Improper documentation:** Failing to record or misrecording what was given.

ROOT CAUSES AND CONTRIBUTING FACTORS

- **Illegible or ambiguous medication orders**
- **Look-alike/sound-alike (LASA) drug names**
- **Interruptions during medication preparation or administration**
- **Lack of familiarity with the drug or its dosing**
- **Fatigue, stress, or high workload**
- **Incomplete patient information (e.g., allergies, labs, renal function)**
- **Poor communication within the healthcare team**

STRATEGIES FOR PREVENTION

1. FOLLOW THE RIGHTS OF MEDICATION ADMINISTRATION

Strictly applying the "10 Rights" consistently is a frontline defense against most errors.

2. USE BARCODE MEDICATION ADMINISTRATION (BCMA)

Barcoding systems reduce errors by ensuring the medication, dose, time, and patient match the MAR.

3. AVOID DISTRACTIONS

Implement no-interruption zones or wear vests signaling medication administration to reduce interruptions during preparation.

4. CLARIFY AND CONFIRM ORDERS

Never guess unclear medication orders. Contact the prescriber or pharmacy for clarification before proceeding.

5. PERFORM INDEPENDENT DOUBLE CHECKS

Especially for high-alert drugs (e.g., insulin, anticoagulants, opioids), have another qualified nurse verify the medication, dose, and route.

6. USE STANDARDIZED PROTOCOLS AND ORDER SETS

Rely on evidence-based protocols to reduce variability and risk in drug selection and administration.

7. REPORT AND ANALYZE ERRORS

Encourage a culture of safety by reporting all medication errors and near-misses through proper channels. Use root cause analysis (RCA) to identify systemic issues.

8. KEEP DRUG KNOWLEDGE CURRENT

Regularly review drug guides, institutional updates, and alerts from the FDA or ISMP. Medication safety requires continuous learning.

TECHNOLOGY AND SAFETY TOOLS

- **Electronic Health Records (EHR):** Helps prevent transcription errors and provides alerts for allergies, interactions, and duplicate therapies.
- **Smart Pumps for IV Medications:** Reduce dosing errors by using pre-programmed drug libraries and limits.
- **Tall-Man Lettering:** Enhances visibility of drug names with similar spellings (e.g., hydrOXYzine vs. hydrALAzine).

NURSING RESPONSIBILITIES

- Ensure safe preparation and labeling of medications.
- Reassess patients after drug administration for any immediate adverse effects.
- Advocate for safety improvements and error prevention training in your unit.
- Engage patients in medication verification whenever appropriate.

CONCLUSION

Preventing medication errors requires a **proactive, systems-based approach** that combines clinical vigilance, teamwork, and standardized safety procedures. Nurses are the final safety check in the medication process and must exercise judgment, precision, and ethical responsibility with every dose administered. By staying informed, minimizing risk factors, and fostering a safety-first culture, medication errors can be significantly reduced—improving outcomes for every patient.

2.5 MONITORING FOR ADVERSE REACTIONS

Adverse drug reactions (ADRs) are unintended, harmful effects that occur at normal therapeutic doses. These reactions can range from mild discomfort to life-threatening events such as anaphylaxis or organ failure. Nurses are in a unique position to identify, monitor, and respond to ADRs due to their close and continuous contact with patients.

Effective monitoring is essential to protect patient safety, prevent complications, and ensure that drug therapy achieves the intended therapeutic outcome.

TYPES OF ADVERSE DRUG REACTIONS

Adverse reactions may present in various forms and timeframes. Common categories include:

- **Type A (Augmented):** Predictable, dose-dependent reactions (e.g., hypoglycemia from insulin).
- **Type B (Bizarre):** Unpredictable, not dose-dependent (e.g., allergic reactions).
- **Acute:** Occur within minutes to hours (e.g., anaphylaxis, arrhythmia).
- **Subacute:** Develop over days (e.g., drug-induced liver injury).
- **Delayed:** Emerge after prolonged use (e.g., tardive dyskinesia from antipsychotics).

COMMON SIGNS OF ADVERSE REACTIONS TO MONITOR

- **Skin:** Rash, hives, itching, flushing, Stevens-Johnson syndrome.
- **Cardiovascular:** Hypotension, tachycardia, arrhythmias.
- **Respiratory:** Dyspnea, bronchospasm, wheezing, stridor.
- **Gastrointestinal:** Nausea, vomiting, diarrhea, GI bleeding.
- **Neurological:** Dizziness, confusion, seizures, tremors.

- **Hematologic:** Bruising, bleeding, pancytopenia.
- **Hepatic/Renal:** Jaundice, dark urine, elevated creatinine, oliguria.

HIGH-RISK DRUG CLASSES FOR ADRS

- **Antibiotics (e.g., penicillins, sulfonamides)** – hypersensitivity, renal toxicity.
- **Opioids** – respiratory depression, constipation, sedation.
- **Anticoagulants** – bleeding, bruising, hematoma.
- **NSAIDs** – GI ulceration, renal impairment.
- **Chemotherapy agents** – bone marrow suppression, mucositis.
- **Psychotropic drugs** – extrapyramidal symptoms, serotonin syndrome.

KEY NURSING RESPONSIBILITIES

1. **Know the Drug**
   - Review each medication's known adverse effects before administration.
   - Understand both common and rare side effects.
2. **Assess the Patient**
   - Perform baseline assessments (vitals, labs, allergy history).
   - Monitor relevant organ systems (e.g., liver enzymes, renal function, ECGs).
3. **Observe and Report**
   - Monitor the patient closely after administration—especially for high-alert or first-time medications.
   - Document changes in physical status, mood, or behavior.
   - Report suspected ADRs to the provider and through internal safety systems.
4. **Respond Appropriately**

- Discontinue the drug (per protocol or prescriber order) if a serious reaction occurs.
- Administer emergency treatments if needed (e.g., epinephrine, oxygen, IV fluids).
- Provide supportive care (e.g., antihistamines, corticosteroids).

5. **Educate the Patient**
    - Instruct patients on what side effects to expect and when to seek medical attention.
    - Encourage reporting of symptoms such as rash, swelling, or difficulty breathing.
    - Document patient teaching and understanding.

DOCUMENTATION TIPS

- Record onset, duration, and severity of symptoms.
- Note the timing of the reaction in relation to drug administration.
- Include vital signs, interventions, and patient outcomes.
- Use standardized reporting tools if applicable (e.g., FDA MedWatch, institutional ADR forms).

SPECIAL CONSIDERATIONS

- **Elderly patients** are more susceptible due to polypharmacy and decreased organ function.
- **Pediatric patients** may be unable to articulate symptoms clearly— observe behavioral changes.
- **Immunocompromised patients** may exhibit atypical or masked reactions.

CONCLUSION

Monitoring for adverse reactions is a core nursing responsibility that requires clinical knowledge, critical thinking, and vigilance. Timely identification and response can be lifesaving and help prevent the progression of minor symptoms into major complications. Nurses should maintain a high index of suspicion for ADRs, especially in high-risk patients or when new medications are introduced.

3. HIGH-ALERT DRUGS & SAFETY WARNINGS

3.1 HIGH-RISK MEDICATIONS (ANTICOAGULANTS, INSULIN, OPIOIDS)

High-risk medications are drugs that carry a **significantly increased risk of causing serious patient harm or death** if used improperly. These medications require **heightened attention, precision, and safety protocols**. Even small errors in dose, timing, or administration can lead to catastrophic outcomes.

Among the most commonly recognized high-risk drug classes in nursing practice are **anticoagulants**, **insulin**, and **opioids**. Each class presents unique challenges that demand thorough understanding and careful handling.

ANTICOAGULANTS

Anticoagulants reduce the blood's ability to clot and are commonly used for conditions such as atrial fibrillation, deep vein thrombosis (DVT), pulmonary embolism (PE), and mechanical heart valves.

Examples:

- Warfarin (Coumadin)
- Heparin (unfractionated)
- Enoxaparin (Lovenox)
- Apixaban (Eliquis)
- Rivaroxaban (Xarelto)
- Dabigatran (Pradaxa)

Risks:

- Internal bleeding

- Intracranial hemorrhage
- Hematuria, GI bleeding
- Drug-drug and drug-food interactions (especially with warfarin)

Nursing Considerations:

- Monitor coagulation labs (INR for warfarin; aPTT for heparin).
- Use weight-based dosing for low-molecular-weight heparins.
- Watch for signs of bleeding (bruising, nosebleeds, bloody stools).
- Educate patients on dietary restrictions and signs of over-anticoagulation.
- Use smart pump technology and double-check protocols.

INSULIN

Insulin is essential for the treatment of type 1 and type 2 diabetes. It is a high-alert drug because errors in type, dose, or timing can lead to **severe hypoglycemia or hyperglycemia**, both of which can be life-threatening.

Types:

- Rapid-acting: Lispro (Humalog), Aspart (NovoLog)
- Short-acting: Regular (Humulin R)
- Intermediate-acting: NPH (Humulin N)
- Long-acting: Glargine (Lantus), Detemir (Levemir)

Risks:

- Hypoglycemia: confusion, tremors, seizures, coma
- Hyperglycemia from missed or insufficient dosing
- Mixing errors (e.g., regular and NPH in wrong order)

Nursing Considerations:

- Use only insulin syringes for measurement.
- Always verify insulin type and dose—especially sliding scale or correctional orders.
- Double-check with a second nurse before administration.
- Monitor blood glucose levels before and after administration.
- Be aware of meal timing relative to insulin type (e.g., rapid-acting should coincide with food intake).
- Know hospital protocols for managing hypoglycemia.

OPIOIDS

Opioids are used for moderate to severe pain management but carry a high risk of **respiratory depression, overdose, and dependence**. Dosing errors, especially in opioid-naïve patients, can be fatal.

Examples:

- Morphine
- Hydromorphone (Dilaudid)
- Fentanyl
- Oxycodone
- Methadone

Risks:

- Respiratory depression and hypoxia
- Sedation and confusion
- Constipation and urinary retention
- Tolerance, dependence, and potential for misuse

Nursing Considerations:

- Assess respiratory rate, sedation level, and pain score before and after administration.

- Use lowest effective dose, especially in elderly and opioid-naïve patients.
- Be cautious with IV opioids—effects may be immediate and profound.
- Always have naloxone (Narcan) available per protocol.
- Educate patients on safe use, side effects, and the importance of not combining opioids with CNS depressants (e.g., benzodiazepines or alcohol).

GENERAL SAFETY STRATEGIES FOR HIGH-RISK MEDICATIONS

- Store high-alert medications in separate, clearly labeled areas.
- Use **tall-man lettering** (e.g., hydrOXYzine vs. hydrALAzine).
- Employ **barcode scanning systems** for medication verification.
- Implement **independent double checks** for all high-alert drugs.
- Use **standardized order sets and protocols** to reduce variation.
- Document administration promptly and monitor closely post-dose.

3.2 BLACK BOX WARNINGS: WHAT NURSES NEED TO KNOW

A **Black Box Warning** (also known as a **Boxed Warning**) is the **strictest warning** issued by the U.S. Food and Drug Administration (FDA) for prescription medications. It appears prominently at the top of a drug's prescribing information, enclosed in a bold black border. These warnings are used to highlight **serious or life-threatening risks** based on clinical evidence, post-marketing surveillance, or safety reports.

Nurses must be aware of these warnings when administering medications to ensure **patient safety**, conduct proper assessments, and provide effective **patient education**.

WHY BLACK BOX WARNINGS MATTER IN NURSING PRACTICE

- Black Box Warnings often indicate **risks that may not be obvious** during routine administration.
- They may **limit how or when a drug is used** (e.g., pregnancy risk, renal failure).
- They frequently require **patient consent**, enhanced monitoring, or **specific protocols**.
- Nurses are often the **first to detect signs** of the adverse effects referenced in these warnings.

COMMON EXAMPLES OF BLACK BOX WARNINGS

1. ANTIDEPRESSANTS (SSRIS, SNRIS, TRICYCLICS)

- **Warning:** Increased risk of suicidal thoughts in children, adolescents, and young adults.
- **Nursing Role:** Monitor mood changes, assess for suicidal ideation, educate family members, and ensure follow-up care.

2. ANTIPSYCHOTICS (E.G., HALOPERIDOL, OLANZAPINE)

- **Warning:** Increased mortality in elderly patients with dementia-related psychosis.
- **Nursing Role:** Evaluate risks and benefits, monitor cognition and behavior, avoid use unless clearly indicated.

3. OPIOIDS (E.G., MORPHINE, FENTANYL, METHADONE)

- **Warning:** Risk of addiction, abuse, misuse, respiratory depression, and death.
- **Nursing Role:** Assess pain appropriately, monitor for overdose symptoms, use lowest effective dose, and educate about safe use.

4. FLUOROQUINOLONES (E.G., CIPROFLOXACIN, LEVOFLOXACIN)

- **Warning:** Tendon rupture, peripheral neuropathy, CNS effects.
- **Nursing Role:** Instruct patient to report tendon pain immediately, avoid in patients with myasthenia gravis.

5. WARFARIN

- **Warning:** Risk of major or fatal bleeding.
- **Nursing Role:** Monitor INR closely, assess for signs of bleeding, and educate patients on drug-food interactions.

6. ISOTRETINOIN (ACCUTANE)

- **Warning:** Extremely high risk of birth defects.
- **Nursing Role:** Ensure strict pregnancy prevention program compliance (iPLEDGE), verify negative pregnancy tests before prescribing or administering.

7. TNF INHIBITORS (E.G., INFLIXIMAB, ADALIMUMAB)

- **Warning:** Risk of serious infections and malignancies.
- **Nursing Role:** Screen for tuberculosis and monitor for signs of infection during therapy.

HOW NURSES CAN IDENTIFY DRUGS WITH BLACK BOX WARNINGS

- Review the **prescribing information** or drug monograph.
- Refer to up-to-date resources like the **FDA website**, institutional drug guides, or the **Institute for Safe Medication Practices (ISMP)**.
- Use drug reference tools with flagged alerts for BBWs (e.g., Davis's Drug Guide, Epocrates, Micromedex).

NURSING RESPONSIBILITIES RELATED TO BBWS

1. **Assessment**
    - Evaluate if the patient has any conditions or risk factors that increase vulnerability to the adverse event described in the warning.
2. **Monitoring**
    - Know which **labs, vital signs, or physical symptoms** to monitor based on the drug's risk profile.
3. **Education**
    - Clearly explain the nature of the warning in layman's terms.
    - Instruct patients to report warning signs (e.g., tendon pain, depression, bleeding).
4. **Documentation**
    - Note any patient teaching, monitoring, or interventions related to the BBW.
    - Document informed refusal or consent when required.
5. **Communication**
    - Collaborate with providers and pharmacists if a drug with a BBW is prescribed to a high-risk patient.
    - Advocate for safer alternatives when appropriate.

3.3 RISK REDUCTION STRATEGIES

In the context of medication administration, **risk reduction strategies** are proactive methods designed to minimize the potential for medication errors, adverse drug events (ADEs), and patient harm—especially when handling **high-alert medications**. Nurses are essential agents in risk management, as they serve as the final checkpoint in the medication delivery process.

This section outlines practical, evidence-based strategies nurses can apply to reduce medication-related risks in every care setting.

1. IMPLEMENT THE "10 RIGHTS" OF MEDICATION ADMINISTRATION

The consistent use of the "10 Rights" (Right patient, drug, dose, route, time, documentation, reason, response, education, and right to refuse) provides a foundational safety net to catch potential errors before they reach the patient.

2. STANDARDIZE HIGH-RISK MEDICATION HANDLING

High-alert medications (e.g., insulin, heparin, opioids) require special handling procedures:

- Use **distinct labeling**, color-coded bins, or tall-man lettering to differentiate look-alike/sound-alike drugs.
- Apply **pre-mixed or pharmacy-prepared solutions** whenever possible.
- Require **independent double checks** for preparation and administration.
- Store separately in clearly designated areas with restricted access.

3. USE TECHNOLOGY SAFELY AND CONSISTENTLY

- **Barcoded Medication Administration (BCMA):** Ensures correct match between patient, drug, and order.
- **Smart IV Pumps:** Allow for pre-programmed drug libraries and dose-limiting safeguards.
- **Electronic Health Records (EHRs):** Enable access to complete medication histories, allergy alerts, and drug interaction warnings.

Technology is a support tool—not a substitute—for clinical judgment.

4. AVOID INTERRUPTIONS DURING MEDICATION PREPARATION

Distractions are a significant source of error. Nurses should:

- Use designated **"No Interruption Zones"** during med prep.
- Avoid engaging in unrelated tasks or conversations when preparing or administering medications.
- Advocate for unit-wide policies that protect concentration during high-risk tasks.

5. CLARIFY ALL MEDICATION ORDERS

- Do not assume intent—always clarify illegible, incomplete, or ambiguous orders.
- Be aware of **decimal point placement** (e.g., "1.0 mg" vs "10 mg"; ".5 mg" vs "0.5 mg").
- Confirm verbal or telephone orders with read-back protocols.

6. MONITOR AND REPORT ADVERSE EVENTS PROMPTLY

- Recognize early signs of adverse drug reactions and toxicity.
- Know how to activate **rapid response protocols**.
- Report adverse events and near misses using your facility's incident reporting system.

Open reporting promotes a culture of safety and learning.

7. ENGAGE IN ONGOING EDUCATION AND SIMULATION

- Stay updated with institutional safety guidelines, national alerts (e.g., FDA, ISMP), and medication recalls.
- Participate in **skills simulations** focused on high-risk medications and critical thinking.
- Complete annual competency validations for IV therapy, chemotherapy, and emergency drug protocols.

8. PROVIDE CLEAR AND CONSISTENT PATIENT EDUCATION

- Educate patients on what medications they are receiving and why.
- Explain how to take medications safely at home, including timing, storage, and what side effects to watch for.
- Empower patients to be active participants in their care by encouraging questions and medication reconciliation.

9. FOSTER INTERDISCIPLINARY COMMUNICATION

- Collaborate with pharmacists and providers when medications are unfamiliar or complex.
- Ensure continuity of care through **handoff reports** that include medication updates, reactions, and pending labs.
- Advocate for **clarity in MARs**, especially during transitions of care.

10. SUPPORT A CULTURE OF SAFETY

- Encourage error reporting without fear of punishment.
- Participate in root cause analyses when errors occur to identify system-level improvements.
- Promote a team-based approach where **everyone shares responsibility** for medication safety.

4. DRUG CLASSIFICATIONS: NURSING ESSENTIALS

4.1 – ANTIBIOTICS AND ANTIMICROBIALS (EXTENDED LIST WITH DOSAGES)

Antibiotics are drugs used to treat bacterial infections. The choice of antibiotic depends on the pathogen,
site of infection, and patient characteristics. Nurses must be aware of spectrum of activity, side effects,
dosage ranges, and key nursing implications.

PENICILLINS

Amoxicillin (Amoxil)
Indications: Streptococcal infections, otitis media, sinusitis, pneumonia
Adult Dose: 500 mg every 8 hours or 875 mg every 12 hours orally
Side Effects: Rash, diarrhea, nausea, allergic reactions (anaphylaxis possible)
Nursing Considerations: Monitor for allergies, give with food if GI upset, complete full course
Penicillin G
Indications: Syphilis, streptococcal infections
Adult Dose: 2.4 million units IM once (syphilis); IV dosing varies
Precautions: Cross-reactivity with cephalosporins (~10%)
Nursing Considerations: Monitor for allergic reactions, rotate IM sites

CEPHALOSPORINS

Cephalexin (Keflex)
Indications: Skin and soft tissue infections, respiratory infections
Adult Dose: 250–500 mg every 6 hours orally
Side Effects: GI upset, rash, candidiasis
Nursing Considerations: Use cautiously in penicillin-allergic patients

Ceftriaxone (Rocephin)
Indications: Pneumonia, gonorrhea, meningitis
Adult Dose: 1–2 g IV/IM daily or divided twice daily
Precautions: Pain at injection site, biliary sludging
Nursing Considerations: Do not mix with calcium-containing solutions in neonates

MACROLIDES

Azithromycin (Zithromax)
Indications: Respiratory infections, STIs (chlamydia)
Adult Dose: 500 mg on day 1, then 250 mg daily on days 2–5
Side Effects: Nausea, diarrhea, QT prolongation
Nursing Considerations: Monitor ECG if risk factors present
Erythromycin
Indications: Acne, pertussis, respiratory infections
Adult Dose: 250–500 mg every 6–12 hours orally
Precautions: Hepatotoxicity, drug interactions
Nursing Considerations: Give on empty stomach if tolerated

TETRACYCLINES

Doxycycline (Vibramycin)
Indications: Acne, Lyme disease, chlamydia, malaria prevention
Adult Dose: 100 mg every 12 hours
Side Effects: Photosensitivity, GI upset
Nursing Considerations: Avoid dairy and antacids; full glass of water**Fluoroquinolones**
Ciprofloxacin (Cipro)
Indications: UTIs, traveler's diarrhea, anthrax
Adult Dose: 250–750 mg orally every 12 hours
Side Effects: Tendon rupture, CNS effects
Nursing Considerations: Avoid calcium/iron; report tendon pain

ANTIFUNGALS

Fluconazole (Diflucan)
Indications: Candidiasis, oral thrush, systemic fungal infections
Adult Dose: 150 mg orally once (vaginal candidiasis) or 200–400 mg/day for systemic infections
Side Effects: Hepatotoxicity, headache, GI upset
Nursing Considerations: Monitor LFTs for prolonged use

ANTIVIRALS

Acyclovir (Zovirax)
Indications: Herpes simplex, shingles, varicella
Adult Dose: 400 mg orally 3–5 times daily or 5–10 mg/kg IV every 8 hours
Side Effects: Nausea, renal toxicity (especially IV)
Nursing Considerations: Encourage hydration; monitor renal function

NURSING SUMMARY
- Always check allergies before administration
- Educate patient to complete the full course
- Monitor for superinfections and adverse reactions
- Assess renal/hepatic function when indicated

SULFONAMIDES
Trimethoprim-Sulfamethoxazole (Bactrim, Septra)
Indications: UTIs, bronchitis, Pneumocystis pneumonia
Adult Dose: 800/160 mg orally every 12 hours
Side Effects: Rash, hyperkalemia, photosensitivity, Stevens-Johnson syndrome
Nursing Considerations: Ensure adequate hydration; monitor for rash and CBC

AMINOGLYCOSIDES
Gentamicin
Indications: Serious gram-negative infections, sepsis
Adult Dose: 3–5 mg/kg/day IV/IM divided every 8 hours
Side Effects: Nephrotoxicity, ototoxicity
Nursing Considerations: Monitor peak/trough levels, renal function, hearing

CARBAPENEMS
Meropenem (Merrem)
Indications: Intra-abdominal infections, meningitis, sepsis
Adult Dose: 500 mg to 1 g IV every 8 hours
Side Effects: Diarrhea, seizures, allergic reactions
Nursing Considerations: Use with caution in CNS disorders; monitor for seizures

LINCOSAMIDESCLINDAMYCIN (CLEOCIN)
Indications: Skin/soft tissue infections, dental infections, anaerobic infections

Adult Dose: 300–450 mg orally every 6–8 hours; 600–900 mg IV every 8 hours
Side Effects: Diarrhea, C. difficile-associated colitis
Nursing Considerations: Monitor for diarrhea; report persistent GI symptoms

NITROFURAN DERIVATIVES

Nitrofurantoin (Macrobid)
Indications: Uncomplicated UTIs
Adult Dose: 100 mg orally twice daily for 5–7 days
Side Effects: GI upset, pulmonary toxicity (rare), urine discoloration

Nursing Considerations: Contraindicated in renal failure; educate on urine color

4.2 – CARDIOVASCULAR DRUGS (EXTENDED, 70+ DRUGS)

ACE INHIBITORS

- Lisinopril (Zestril, Prinivil)

Indications: HTN, HF, post-MI

Dose: 10–40 mg once daily

Side Effects: Dry cough, hyperkalemia, angioedema

Nursing Considerations: Monitor K+, BP, renal function

- Enalapril (Vasotec)

Indications: HTN, HF

Dose: 5–20 mg/day

Side Effects: Same as above

Nursing Considerations: Monitor labs

- Ramipril (Altace)

Indications: HTN, post-MI

Dose: 2.5–10 mg/day

Side Effects: Cough, hypotension

Nursing Considerations: Watch for orthostatic hypotension

- Perindopril (Aceon)

Indications: HTN

Dose: 4–16 mg/day

Side Effects: Hyperkalemia

Nursing Considerations: Monitor electrolytes

ARBS

- Losartan (Cozaar)

Indications: HTN, diabetic nephropathy

Dose: 25–100 mg/day

Side Effects: Hyperkalemia

Nursing Considerations: Monitor renal function

- Valsartan (Diovan)

Indications: HTN, HF

Dose: 80–320 mg/day

Side Effects: Dizziness, renal dysfunction

Nursing Considerations: Monitor BUN/Cr

- Olmesartan (Benicar)

Indications: HTN

Dose: 20–40 mg/day

Side Effects: GI upset

Nursing Considerations: Watch for hypotension

- Telmisartan (Micardis)

Indications: HTN

Dose: 20–80 mg/day

Side Effects: Fatigue

Nursing Considerations: Check BP regularly

BETA BLOCKERS
- Metoprolol (Lopressor)

Indications: HTN, angina, HF

Dose: 50–100 mg BID

Side Effects: Bradycardia, fatigue

Nursing Considerations: Hold if HR <60

- Atenolol (Tenormin)

Indications: HTN, angina

Dose: 25–100 mg/day

Side Effects: Cold extremities

Nursing Considerations: Monitor HR

- Carvedilol (Coreg)

Indications: HF

Dose: 6.25–25 mg BID

Side Effects: Hypotension

Nursing Considerations: Take with food

- Propranolol (Inderal)

Indications: HTN, anxiety

Dose: 40–160 mg/day

Side Effects: Depression

Nursing Considerations: Caution in asthma

- Nadolol (Corgard)

Indications: HTN, angina

Dose: 40–320 mg/day

Side Effects: Fatigue

Nursing Considerations: Long half-life

- Labetalol (Trandate)

Indications: HTN, HTN emergency

Dose: 100–400 mg BID

Side Effects: Orthostatic hypotension

Nursing Considerations: Check BP frequently

- Esmolol (Brevibloc)

Indications: SVT, intraop control

Dose: IV infusion

Side Effects: Bradycardia

Nursing Considerations: Continuous monitoring

CALCIUM CHANNEL BLOCKERS
- Amlodipine (Norvasc)

Indications: HTN, angina

Dose: 5–10 mg/day

Side Effects: Peripheral edema

Nursing Considerations: Monitor for swelling

- Diltiazem (Cardizem)

Indications: AFib, HTN

Dose: 180–360 mg/day

Side Effects: Bradycardia

Nursing Considerations: Check HR

- Verapamil (Calan)

Indications: HTN, arrhythmia

Dose: 120–480 mg/day

Side Effects: Constipation

Nursing Considerations: Encourage fluids

DIURETICS
- HCTZ

Indications: HTN, fluid retention

Dose: 12.5–50 mg/day

Side Effects: Hypokalemia

Nursing Considerations: Monitor electrolytes

- Furosemide (Lasix)

Indications: Edema, CHF

Dose: 20–80 mg/day

Side Effects: Ototoxicity

Nursing Considerations: Daily weights

- Bumetanide (Bumex)

Indications: CHF

Dose: 0.5–2 mg/day

Side Effects: Dehydration

Nursing Considerations: Monitor I&O

- Spironolactone (Aldactone)

Indications: HF, ascites

Dose: 25–100 mg/day

Side Effects: Hyperkalemia, gynecomastia

Nursing Considerations: Avoid K+ supplements

- Eplerenone (Inspra)

Indications: HTN, post-MI

Dose: 25–50 mg/day

Side Effects: Less endocrine SE

Nursing Considerations: Monitor K+

ANTICOAGULANTS
- Warfarin (Coumadin)

Indications: AFib, DVT

Dose: 2–10 mg/day

Side Effects: Bleeding

Nursing Considerations: Monitor INR

- Heparin

Indications: VTE treatment

Dose: IV based on aPTT

Side Effects: HIT

Nursing Considerations: Check platelets

- Enoxaparin (Lovenox)

Indications: DVT prophylaxis

Dose: 40 mg SC daily

Side Effects: Injection site bruising

Nursing Considerations: Don't expel air bubble

- Rivaroxaban (Xarelto)

Indications: DVT, stroke prevention

Dose: 10–20 mg/day

Side Effects: Bleeding

Nursing Considerations: Take with food

- Apixaban (Eliquis)

Indications: AFib, DVT

Dose: 5 mg BID

Side Effects: GI bleeding

Nursing Considerations: Monitor signs of bleeding

- Dabigatran (Pradaxa)

Indications: Stroke prevention

Dose: 150 mg BID

Side Effects: GI discomfort

Nursing Considerations: Keep in original bottle

ANTIPLATELETS

- Aspirin (ASA)

Indications: MI prevention

Dose: 81–325 mg/day

Side Effects: GI ulcers

Nursing Considerations: Take with food

- Clopidogrel (Plavix)

Indications: Post-stent, stroke

Dose: 75 mg/day

Side Effects: Bruising

Nursing Considerations: Avoid NSAIDs

- Ticagrelor (Brilinta)

Indications: ACS

Dose: 90 mg BID

Side Effects: SOB, bleeding

Nursing Considerations: Monitor adherence

LIPID-LOWERING AGENTS
- Atorvastatin (Lipitor)

Indications: Hyperlipidemia

Dose: 10–80 mg/day

Side Effects: Myopathy, liver enzymes

Nursing Considerations: Avoid grapefruit

- Rosuvastatin (Crestor)

Indications: Hyperlipidemia

Dose: 5–40 mg/day

Side Effects: Muscle pain

Nursing Considerations: Check CK levels

- Simvastatin (Zocor)

Indications: Cholesterol

Dose: 10–40 mg/day

Side Effects: Rhabdomyolysis

Nursing Considerations: Take in evening

- Ezetimibe (Zetia)

Indications: Cholesterol

Dose: 10 mg/day

Side Effects: GI upset

Nursing Considerations: Used with statins

- Fenofibrate (Tricor)

Indications: Triglycerides

Dose: 48–145 mg/day

Side Effects: Gallstones

Nursing Considerations: Monitor LFTs

ANTIARRHYTHMICS
- Amiodarone (Cordarone)

Indications: Ventricular arrhythmias

Dose: 200–400 mg/day

Side Effects: Thyroid/lung toxicity

Nursing Considerations: Baseline labs, ECG

Dose: 0.125–0.25 mg/day

Side Effects: N/V, visual changes

Nursing Considerations: Check apical pulse, level

- Sotalol (Betapace)

Indications: AFib

Dose: 80–160 mg BID

Side Effects: QT prolongation

Nursing Considerations: Monitor ECG

- Hydralazine

Indications: HTN

Dose: 10–50 mg QID

Side Effects: Lupus-like syndrome

Nursing Considerations: Monitor ANA if long term

- Lidocaine (Xylocaine)

Indications: Ventricular arrhythmia

Dose: IV bolus/infusion

Side Effects: Neurotoxicity

Nursing Considerations: ICU monitoring

- Isosorbide Mononitrate (Imdur)

Indications: Angina

Dose: 30–120 mg/day

Side Effects: Headache

Nursing Considerations: Do not crush

OTHER CARDIOVASCULAR MEDICATIONS

- Digoxin (Lanoxin)

Indications: HF, AFib

- Nitroglycerin (Nitrostat)

Indications: Angina (acute)

Dose: 0.3–0.6 mg SL q5min x3

Side Effects: Hypotension

Nursing Considerations: Sit before taking

- Dobutamine

Indications: Acute HF

Dose: IV infusion

Side Effects: Tachycardia

Nursing Considerations: ICU setting

- Milrinone

Indications: Cardiogenic shock

Dose: IV infusion

Side Effects: Hypotension

Nursing Considerations: Continuous BP monitoring

Dose: IV infusion

Side Effects: Cyanide toxicity

Nursing Considerations: Protect from light

- Norepinephrine (Levophed)

Indications: Shock

Dose: IV titrated

Side Effects: Bradycardia, vasoconstriction

Nursing Considerations: Central line preferred

- Nitroprusside (Nipride)

Indications: HTN crisis

4.3 Analgesics & Anti-Inflammatories
4.4 CNS Medications (Psychiatric, Seizure, Sleep)
4.5 Endocrine & Metabolic Agents
4.6 Gastrointestinal Medications
4.7 Respiratory Medications
4.8 Immune System Agents
4.9 Renal & Urinary Drugs
4.10 Reproductive Health Medications

4.3 – ANALGESICS AND ANTI-INFLAMMATORY DRUGS (EXTENDED LIST)

NON-STEROIDAL ANTI-INFLAMMATORY DRUGS (NSAIDS)

- Ibuprofen (Advil, Motrin)

Indications: Mild to moderate pain, fever, inflammation

Dose: 200–800 mg every 6–8 hours

Side Effects: GI bleeding, renal impairment

Nursing Considerations: Take with food

Indications: Moderate to severe pain

Dose: 15–30 mg IV/IM q6h (max 5 days)

Side Effects: Nephrotoxicity, GI risk

Nursing Considerations: Short-term only

- Diclofenac (Voltaren)

Indications: Arthritis, pain

Dose: 50 mg BID-TID

- Naproxen (Aleve, Naprosyn)

Indications: Pain, arthritis

Dose: 250–500 mg twice daily

Side Effects: GI upset, bleeding risk

Nursing Considerations: Avoid in ulcers

- Ketorolac (Toradol)

Side Effects: GI discomfort, liver issues

Nursing Considerations: Topical and oral forms

- Indomethacin (Indocin)

Indications: Gout, arthritis

Dose: 25–50 mg BID-TID

Side Effects: Peptic ulcers, headache

Nursing Considerations: Short-term use

- Meloxicam (Mobic)

Indications: Osteoarthritis

Dose: 7.5–15 mg daily

Side Effects: GI bleeding

Nursing Considerations: Once daily

- Celecoxib (Celebrex)

Indications: Arthritis, dysmenorrhea

Dose: 100–200 mg BID

Side Effects: Thrombosis risk

Nursing Considerations: Less GI side effects

- Etodolac

Indications: Pain, osteoarthritis

Dose: 200–400 mg every 6–8 hrs

Side Effects: GI discomfort

Nursing Considerations: Take with food

- Piroxicam (Feldene)

Indications: Rheumatoid arthritis

Dose: 10–20 mg/day

Side Effects: GI and renal toxicity

Nursing Considerations: Not first-line

- Sulindac

Indications: Pain, inflammation

Dose: 150–200 mg BID

Side Effects: GI side effects

Nursing Considerations: Monitor renal function

OPIOID ANALGESICS

- Morphine

Indications: Severe pain

Dose: 2–10 mg IV or 15–30 mg PO q4h

Side Effects: Respiratory depression

Nursing Considerations: Monitor RR and sedation

- Hydromorphone (Dilaudid)

Indications: Severe pain

Dose: 0.2–1 mg IV q2–3h

Side Effects: Sedation, hypotension

Nursing Considerations: Potent opioid

- Oxycodone

Indications: Moderate to severe pain

Dose: 5–15 mg PO q4–6h

Side Effects: Constipation, nausea

Nursing Considerations: May combine with acetaminophen

- Hydrocodone/Acetaminophen

Indications: Moderate pain

Dose: 5/325 to 10/325 mg q4–6h

Side Effects: Liver toxicity

Nursing Considerations: Limit daily acetaminophen

- Fentanyl

Indications: Severe pain

Dose: 25–100 mcg IV or patch q72h

Side Effects: Respiratory depression

Nursing Considerations: Only for opioid-tolerant

- Codeine

Indications: Mild to moderate pain

Dose: 15–60 mg q4–6h

Side Effects: Sedation, nausea

Nursing Considerations: Also used as antitussive

- Tramadol

Indications: Moderate pain

Dose: 50–100 mg q4–6h (max 400 mg/day)

Side Effects: Seizure risk, dizziness

Nursing Considerations: Lower abuse potential

- Tapentadol (Nucynta)

Indications: Moderate to severe pain

Dose: 50–100 mg q4–6h

Side Effects: Nausea, sedation

Nursing Considerations: Dual-action analgesic

- Methadone

Indications: Chronic pain, opioid detox

Dose: 2.5–10 mg q8–12h

Side Effects: QT prolongation

Nursing Considerations: Long half-life

- Buprenorphine

Indications: Pain, opioid dependence

Dose: 2–8 mg SL

Side Effects: Ceiling effect

Nursing Considerations: Monitor for withdrawal symptoms

ACETAMINOPHEN

- Acetaminophen (Tylenol)

Indications: Fever, mild pain

Dose: 325–1000 mg q4–6h (max 4g/day)

Side Effects: Hepatotoxicity

Nursing Considerations: Monitor liver function

- Acetaminophen/Codeine (Tylenol #3)

Indications: Moderate pain

Dose: 1–2 tablets q4–6h

Side Effects: Drowsiness, constipation

Nursing Considerations: Schedule III drug

CORTICOSTEROIDS

- Prednisone

Indications: Inflammatory diseases

Dose: 5–60 mg/day

Side Effects: Hyperglycemia, weight gain

Nursing Considerations: Taper gradually

- Methylprednisolone (Solu-Medrol)

Indications: Acute inflammation

Dose: 10–80 mg/day IV or PO

Side Effects: Immunosuppression

Nursing Considerations: Avoid long-term use

- Dexamethasone

Indications: Edema, inflammation

Dose: 4–20 mg/day

Side Effects: Mood changes, insomnia

Nursing Considerations: Long-acting steroid

- Hydrocortisone

Indications: Adrenal insufficiency

Dose: 15–240 mg/day

Side Effects: Cushingoid features

Nursing Considerations: Monitor glucose

MISCELLANEOUS ANALGESICS

- Ketamine

Indications: Procedural sedation, pain

Dose: 0.1–0.5 mg/kg IV

Side Effects: Hallucinations, HTN

Nursing Considerations: Monitor cardiac and mental status

- Lidocaine

Indications: Local anesthesia, neuropathic pain

Dose: Topical or IV

Side Effects: CNS toxicity

Nursing Considerations: Cardiac monitoring if IV

- Gabapentin (Neurontin)

Indications: Neuropathic pain

Dose: 300–1800 mg/day

Side Effects: Dizziness, sedation

Nursing Considerations: Start low, titrate up

- Pregabalin (Lyrica)

Indications: Neuropathy, fibromyalgia

Dose: 150–600 mg/day

Side Effects: Weight gain, dizziness

Nursing Considerations: Controlled substance

- Capsaicin (Zostrix)

Indications: Arthritis, neuralgia

Dose: Topical application

Side Effects: Burning sensation

Nursing Considerations: Wash hands after use

- Carbamazepine (Tegretol)

Indications: Neuropathic pain

Dose: 200–1200 mg/day

Side Effects: Drowsiness, hyponatremia

Nursing Considerations: Monitor sodium

- Valproic Acid (Depakote)

Indications: Migraine prevention

Dose: 250–1000 mg/day

Side Effects: Tremor, weight gain

Nursing Considerations: Liver enzyme monitoring

- Amitriptyline

Indications: Chronic pain, neuropathy

Dose: 10–75 mg at bedtime

Side Effects: Dry mouth, sedation

Nursing Considerations: Orthostatic precautions

- Nortriptyline

Indications: Neuropathic pain

Dose: 25–75 mg/day

Side Effects: Anticholinergic effects

Nursing Considerations: Titrate slowly

- Baclofen

Indications: Muscle spasms

Dose: 5–20 mg TID

Side Effects: Sedation, weakness

Nursing Considerations: Do not stop abruptly

4.4 – CENTRAL NERVOUS SYSTEM MEDICATIONS (EXTENDED LIST).

ANTIDEPRESSANTS – SSRIS, SNRIS, TCAS, MAOIS

- Fluoxetine (Prozac)

Indications: Depression, anxiety

Dose: 10–80 mg/day

Side Effects: Insomnia, GI upset

Nursing Considerations: Take in morning

- Sertraline (Zoloft)

Indications: Depression, PTSD

Dose: 25–200 mg/day

Side Effects: Sexual dysfunction, nausea

Nursing Considerations: Monitor mood

- Paroxetine (Paxil)

Indications: Depression, anxiety

Dose: 20–50 mg/day

Side Effects: Sedation, weight gain

Nursing Considerations: Taper off slowly

- Citalopram (Celexa)

Indications: Depression

Dose: 20–40 mg/day

Side Effects: QT prolongation

Nursing Considerations: Check ECG in elderly

- Escitalopram (Lexapro)

Indications: Anxiety, depression

Dose: 10–20 mg/day

Side Effects: Drowsiness

Nursing Considerations: Onset: 1–4 weeks

- Duloxetine (Cymbalta)

Indications: Depression, neuropathy

Dose: 30–120 mg/day

Side Effects: Dry mouth, fatigue

Nursing Considerations: Monitor liver function

- Venlafaxine (Effexor)

Indications: Depression, panic disorder

Dose: 75–225 mg/day

Side Effects: Hypertension

Nursing Considerations: Check BP regularly

- Amitriptyline (Elavil)

Indications: Chronic pain, depression

Dose: 25–150 mg/day

Side Effects: Anticholinergic effects

Nursing Considerations: Take at bedtime

- Nortriptyline (Pamelor)

Indications: Neuropathy, depression

Dose: 25–100 mg/day

Side Effects: Sedation

Nursing Considerations: Monitor ECG

- Phenelzine (Nardil)

Indications: Depression (MAOI)

Dose: 15–90 mg/day

Side Effects: HTN crisis with tyramine

Nursing Considerations: Avoid aged foods

ANTIPSYCHOTICS – TYPICAL AND ATYPICAL

- Haloperidol (Haldol)

Indications: Schizophrenia, agitation

Dose: 2–20 mg/day

Side Effects: EPS, sedation

Nursing Considerations: Monitor for dystonia

- Chlorpromazine (Thorazine)

Indications: Psychosis, nausea

Dose: 25–400 mg/day

Side Effects: Orthostatic hypotension

Nursing Considerations: Fall precautions

- Risperidone (Risperdal)

Indications: Schizophrenia, bipolar

Dose: 1–8 mg/day

Side Effects: Weight gain, EPS

Nursing Considerations: Monitor prolactin

- Olanzapine (Zyprexa)

Indications: Bipolar, schizophrenia

Dose: 5–20 mg/day

Side Effects: Metabolic syndrome

Nursing Considerations: Check glucose/lipids

- Quetiapine (Seroquel)

Indications: Depression, psychosis

Dose: 150–800 mg/day

Side Effects: Sedation

Nursing Considerations: Monitor mood/weight

- Aripiprazole (Abilify)

Indications: Depression adjunct, psychosis

Dose: 10–30 mg/day

Side Effects: Akathisia

Nursing Considerations: Monitor for agitation

- Ziprasidone (Geodon)

Indications: Bipolar, schizophrenia

Dose: 20–160 mg/day

Side Effects: QT prolongation

Nursing Considerations: Give with food

- Lurasidone (Latuda)

Indications: Schizophrenia

Dose: 40–160 mg/day

Side Effects: Nausea, somnolence

Nursing Considerations: Take with food

- Paliperidone (Invega)

Indications: Schizophrenia

Dose: 3–12 mg/day

Side Effects: EPS, increased prolactin

Nursing Considerations: Monitor renal function

- Clozapine (Clozaril)

Indications: Resistant schizophrenia

Dose: 100–900 mg/day

Side Effects: Agranulocytosis

Nursing Considerations: Weekly CBCs

ANTIEPILEPTICS / ANTICONVULSANTS

- Phenytoin (Dilantin)

Indications: Seizures

Dose: 300–400 mg/day

Side Effects: Gingival hyperplasia

Nursing Considerations: Monitor serum levels

- Carbamazepine (Tegretol)

Indications: Seizures, bipolar

Dose: 200–1200 mg/day

Side Effects: Hyponatremia

Nursing Considerations: Monitor sodium

- Valproic acid (Depakote)

Indications: Seizures, mood

Dose: 500–2000 mg/day

Side Effects: Hepatotoxicity

Nursing Considerations: Check LFTs

Side Effects: Rash (SJS)

Nursing Considerations: Titrate slowly

- Levetiracetam (Keppra)

Indications: Seizures

Dose: 500–3000 mg/day

Side Effects: Irritability

Nursing Considerations: Monitor mood

- Topiramate (Topamax)

Indications: Seizures, migraines

Dose: 50–400 mg/day

Side Effects: Cognitive dulling

Nursing Considerations: Hydration important

- Lamotrigine (Lamictal)

Indications: Seizures, bipolar

Dose: 25–500 mg/day

- Gabapentin (Neurontin)

Indications: Neuropathy, seizures

Dose: 300–1800 mg/day

Side Effects: Sedation, dizziness

Nursing Considerations: Dose adjust in renal

- Pregabalin (Lyrica)

Indications: Fibromyalgia, seizures

Dose: 150–600 mg/day

Side Effects: Weight gain

Nursing Considerations: Schedule V drug

- Oxcarbazepine (Trileptal)

Indications: Partial seizures

Dose: 600–2400 mg/day

Side Effects: Hyponatremia

Nursing Considerations: Monitor Na+

- Clonazepam (Klonopin)

Indications: Seizures, panic disorder

Dose: 0.5–4 mg/day

Side Effects: Sedation

Nursing Considerations: Avoid abrupt withdrawal

ANXIOLYTICS / SEDATIVES / HYPNOTICS

- Lorazepam (Ativan)

Indications: Anxiety, status epilepticus

Dose: 0.5–4 mg/day

Side Effects: Sedation

Nursing Considerations: Short-acting benzo

- Diazepam (Valium)

Indications: Anxiety, seizures

Dose: 2–10 mg BID-QID

Side Effects: Respiratory depression

Nursing Considerations: Long-acting

- Alprazolam (Xanax)

Indications: Panic disorder

Dose: 0.25–4 mg/day

Side Effects: Dependence

Nursing Considerations: Avoid alcohol

- Clonazepam (Klonopin)

Indications: Panic, seizures

Dose: 0.5–4 mg/day

Side Effects: Drowsiness

Nursing Considerations: Schedule IV

- Buspirone (Buspar)

Indications: Generalized anxiety

Dose: 10–30 mg/day

Side Effects: Dizziness, nausea

Nursing Considerations: Takes weeks to work

- Hydroxyzine (Vistaril)

Indications: Anxiety, itching

Dose: 25–100 mg q6h

Side Effects: Drowsiness

Nursing Considerations: Non-addictive

- Zolpidem (Ambien)

Indications: Insomnia

Dose: 5–10 mg at bedtime

Side Effects: Sleepwalking

Nursing Considerations: Use short-term

- Eszopiclone (Lunesta)

Indications: Insomnia

Dose: 1–3 mg at bedtime

Side Effects: Bitter taste

Nursing Considerations: Monitor for dependence

- Temazepam (Restoril)

Indications: Insomnia

Dose: 7.5–30 mg at bedtime

Side Effects: Daytime drowsiness

Nursing Considerations: Limit to 2 weeks

- Trazodone

Indications: Sleep, depression

Dose: 50–300 mg at bedtime

Side Effects: Sedation, priapism

Nursing Considerations: Often used off-lab

4.5 – ENDOCRINE AND METABOLIC MEDICATIONS (EXTENDED LIST)

INSULINS

- Insulin Regular (Humulin R)

Indications: Type 1 and 2 diabetes

Dose: SQ/IV 0.1 units/kg or sliding scale

Side Effects: Hypoglycemia, weight gain

Nursing Considerations: Check glucose before giving

- Insulin NPH (Humulin N)

Indications: Intermediate-acting insulin

Dose: SQ BID

Side Effects: Hypoglycemia, lipodystrophy

Nursing Considerations: Roll to mix, do not shake

- Insulin Glargine (Lantus)

Indications: Basal insulin

Dose: SQ once daily

Side Effects: No peak, risk of hypoglycemia

Nursing Considerations: Do not mix with other insulins

- Insulin Detemir (Levemir)

Indications: Long-acting insulin

Dose: SQ once or twice daily

Side Effects: Injection site reaction

Nursing Considerations: Use consistent timing

- Insulin Aspart (Novolog)

Indications: Rapid-acting insulin

Dose: SQ at meals

Side Effects: Hypoglycemia

Nursing Considerations: Give 5–10 mins before meal

- Insulin Lispro (Humalog)

- Insulin Degludec (Tresiba)

Indications: Ultra-long-acting insulin

Dose: SQ once daily

Side Effects: Hypoglycemia

Nursing Considerations: Flexible dosing time

ORAL ANTIDIABETICS
- Metformin (Glucophage)

Indications: Type 2 diabetes

Dose: 500–2000 mg/day

Side Effects: GI upset, lactic acidosis

Nursing Considerations: Take with meals, monitor renal function

- Glyburide

Indications: Rapid-acting insulin

Dose: SQ at meals

Side Effects: Hypoglycemia

Nursing Considerations: Monitor glucose closely

Indications: Type 2 diabetes

Dose: 1.25–20 mg/day

Side Effects: Hypoglycemia, weight gain

Nursing Considerations: Caution in elderly

- Glipizide

Indications: Type 2 diabetes

Dose: 2.5–40 mg/day

Side Effects: Hypoglycemia

Nursing Considerations: Take 30 min before meals

- Glimepiride

Indications: Type 2 diabetes

Dose: 1–8 mg/day

Side Effects: Weight gain

Nursing Considerations: Monitor glucose regularly

- Sitagliptin (Januvia)

Indications: Type 2 diabetes

Dose: 100 mg/day

Side Effects: Pancreatitis, nasopharyngitis

Nursing Considerations: Adjust in renal impairment

- Linagliptin (Tradjenta)

Indications: Type 2 diabetes

Dose: 5 mg/day

Side Effects: Joint pain

Nursing Considerations: No renal adjustment needed

- Canagliflozin (Invokana)

Indications: Type 2 diabetes

Dose: 100–300 mg/day

Side Effects: UTIs, DKA

Nursing Considerations: Monitor for genital infections

- Dapagliflozin (Farxiga)

Indications: Type 2 diabetes, HF

Dose: 5–10 mg/day

Side Effects: Volume depletion

Nursing Considerations: Check renal function

- Pioglitazone (Actos)

Indications: Type 2 diabetes

Dose: 15–45 mg/day

Side Effects: Fluid retention, weight gain

Nursing Considerations: Contraindicated in CHF

- Acarbose

Indications: Type 2 diabetes

Dose: 25–100 mg TID

Side Effects: Flatulence, diarrhea

Nursing Considerations: Take with first bite of food

THYROID HORMONES AND ANTAGONISTS

- Levothyroxine (Synthroid)

Indications: Hypothyroidism

Dose: 25–200 mcg/day

Side Effects: Tachycardia, weight loss

Nursing Considerations: Give in AM on empty stomach

- Liothyronine (Cytomel)

Indications: Hypothyroidism

Dose: 25–100 mcg/day

Side Effects: Arrhythmia

Nursing Considerations: Monitor T3 levels

- Propylthiouracil (PTU)

Indications: Hyperthyroidism

Dose: 100–600 mg/day

Side Effects: Hepatotoxicity

Nursing Considerations: Monitor liver enzymes, CBC

- Methimazole (Tapazole)

Indications: Hyperthyroidism

Dose: 5–30 mg/day

Side Effects: Agranulocytosis

Nursing Considerations: Report sore throat, fever

CORTICOSTEROIDS

- Prednisone

Indications: Inflammation, adrenal insufficiency

Dose: 5–60 mg/day

Side Effects: Hyperglycemia, immunosuppression

Nursing Considerations: Taper slowly

- Hydrocortisone

Indications: Adrenal insufficiency

Dose: 15–240 mg/day

Side Effects: Mood changes

Nursing Considerations: Give with food

- Dexamethasone

Indications: Cerebral edema, inflammation

Dose: 4–20 mg/day

Side Effects: Insomnia, hypertension

Nursing Considerations: Use lowest effective dose

- Methylprednisolone (Medrol, Solu-Medrol)

Indications: Autoimmune, asthma

Dose: 10–80 mg/day

Side Effects: Infection risk

Nursing Considerations: Monitor blood sugar

OTHER ENDOCRINE AGENTS
- Desmopressin (DDAVP)

Indications: Diabetes insipidus, bedwetting

Dose: 0.1–0.6 mg/day

Side Effects: Hyponatremia

Nursing Considerations: Monitor sodium levels

- Octreotide (Sandostatin)

Indications: Acromegaly, carcinoid tumors

Dose: 50–1500 mcg/day

Side Effects: GI upset

Nursing Considerations: Check glucose, liver enzymes

- Levothyroxine + Liothyronine (Thyrolar)

Indications: Hypothyroidism

Dose: 1/2–2 tablets daily

Side Effects: Palpitations

Nursing Considerations: Monitor TSH

- Fludrocortisone (Florinef)

Indications: Addison's disease

Dose: 0.1–0.2 mg/day

Side Effects: HTN, edema

Nursing Considerations: Monitor BP and electrolytes

- Cinacalcet (Sensipar)

Indications: Hyperparathyroidism

Dose: 30–180 mg/day

Side Effects: Nausea, hypocalcemia

Nursing Considerations: Monitor calciu

4.6 – GASTROINTESTINAL MEDICATIONS (EXTENDED LIST)

ANTACIDS
- Calcium carbonate (Tums)

Indications: Heartburn, indigestion

Dose: 500–1000 mg as needed

Side Effects: Constipation, hypercalcemia

Nursing Considerations: Avoid excessive use

- Magnesium hydroxide (Milk of Magnesia)

Indications: Heartburn, constipation

Dose: 400–1200 mg/day

Side Effects: Diarrhea

Nursing Considerations: Avoid in renal failure

- Aluminum hydroxide

Indications: Heartburn

Dose: 500–1500 mg/day

Side Effects: Constipation

Nursing Considerations: May cause phosphate depletion

- Sodium bicarbonate

Indications: Indigestion, metabolic acidosis

Dose: 325–2000 mg/day

Side Effects: Alkalosis, gas

Nursing Considerations: Short-term use only

H2 RECEPTOR ANTAGONISTS
- Ranitidine (withdrawn)

Indications: GERD, ulcers

Dose: 150 mg BID

Side Effects: Headache

Nursing Considerations: No longer available in US

- Famotidine (Pepcid)

Indications: GERD, ulcers

Dose: 20–40 mg/day

Side Effects: Constipation, dizziness

Nursing Considerations: Take at bedtime

- Cimetidine (Tagamet)

Indications: GERD

Dose: 300–800 mg BID-QID

Side Effects: Gynecomastia

Nursing Considerations: Many drug interactions

PROTON PUMP INHIBITORS (PPIS)

- Omeprazole (Prilosec)

Indications: GERD, ulcers

Dose: 20–40 mg/day

Side Effects: Headache, B12 deficiency

Nursing Considerations: Take before meals

- Pantoprazole (Protonix)

Indications: GERD, erosive esophagitis

Dose: 20–40 mg/day

Side Effects: Flatulence, nausea

Nursing Considerations: Do not crush

- Esomeprazole (Nexium)

Indications: GERD, ulcers

Dose: 20–40 mg/day

Side Effects: Constipation

Nursing Considerations: Long-term use risk

- Lansoprazole (Prevacid)

Indications: GERD

Dose: 15–30 mg/day

Side Effects: Diarrhea, abdominal pain

Nursing Considerations: Take on empty stomach

- Dexlansoprazole (Dexilant)

Indications: GERD

Dose: 30–60 mg/day

Side Effects: C. diff risk

Nursing Considerations: Extended-release formulation

LAXATIVES AND STOOL SOFTENERS

- Psyllium (Metamucil)

Indications: Constipation

Dose: 3.4–10 g/day

Side Effects: Bloating, gas

Nursing Considerations: Take with full glass of water

- Docusate sodium (Colace)

Indications: Stool softener

Dose: 100–300 mg/day

Side Effects: Mild cramps

Nursing Considerations: Use for prevention

- Senna (Senokot)

Indications: Constipation

Dose: 15–30 mg/day

Side Effects: Abdominal cramping

Nursing Considerations: Use short-term

- Bisacodyl (Dulcolax)

Indications: Bowel prep, constipation

Dose: 5–15 mg/day

Side Effects: Dependency risk

Nursing Considerations: Avoid chronic use

- Lactulose

Indications: Constipation, hepatic encephalopathy

Dose: 15–30 mL/day

Side Effects: Diarrhea, bloating

Nursing Considerations: Monitor ammonia levels

- Polyethylene glycol (MiraLAX)

Indications: Constipation

Dose: 17 g in 8 oz water daily

Side Effects: Flatulence

Nursing Considerations: Well tolerated

- Magnesium citrate

Indications: Bowel prep

Dose: 150–300 mL

Side Effects: Electrolyte imbalance

Nursing Considerations: Rapid onset

ANTIDIARRHEALS
- Loperamide (Imodium)

Indications: Acute diarrhea

Dose: 4 mg initially, then 2 mg after stools

Side Effects: Constipation, dizziness

Nursing Considerations: Do not exceed 8 mg/day OTC

- Diphenoxylate/atropine (Lomotil)

Indications: Diarrhea

Dose: 5 mg 3–4 times/day

Side Effects: Drowsiness, dry mouth

Nursing Considerations: Controlled substance

- Bismuth subsalicylate (Pepto-Bismol)

Indications: Diarrhea, H. pylori

Dose: 524 mg every 30–60 min

Side Effects: Black stools, tinnitus

Nursing Considerations: Avoid in children

ANTIEMETICS
- Ondansetron (Zofran)

Indications: Nausea, vomiting

Dose: 4–8 mg PRN

Side Effects: Headache, QT prolongation

Nursing Considerations: Effective for chemo-induced N/V

- Promethazine (Phenergan)

Indications: Nausea, motion sickness

Dose: 12.5–25 mg q4–6h

Side Effects: Sedation

Nursing Considerations: Monitor for EPS

- Metoclopramide (Reglan)

Indications: N/V, gastroparesis

Dose: 10–15 mg q6–8h

Side Effects: Tardive dyskinesia

Nursing Considerations: Avoid chronic use

- Prochlorperazine (Compazine)

Indications: N/V, psychosis

Dose: 5–10 mg q6–8h

Side Effects: Dystonia

Nursing Considerations: Monitor for EPS

- Scopolamine (Transderm Scop)

Indications: Motion sickness

Dose: 1 patch q72h

Side Effects: Dry mouth, drowsiness

Nursing Considerations: Apply behind ear

- Meclizine (Antivert)

Indications: Vertigo, motion sickness

Dose: 25–100 mg/day

Side Effects: Sedation, dry mouth

Nursing Considerations: OTC option

OTHER GI MEDICATIONS
- Sucralfate (Carafate)

Indications: Ulcers

Dose: 1 g QID before meals

Side Effects: Constipation

Nursing Considerations: Needs acid to activate

- Misoprostol (Cytotec)

Indications: Ulcer prevention (NSAID)

Dose: 200 mcg QID

Side Effects: Diarrhea, uterine contractions

Nursing Considerations: Avoid in pregnancy

- Simethicone (Gas-X)

Indications: Gas relief

Dose: 40–125 mg QID

Side Effects: Very few side effects

Nursing Considerations: Often combined with antacids

- Ursodiol (Actigall)

Indications: Gallstone dissolution

Dose: 300 mg BID

Side Effects: Diarrhea, back pain

Nursing Considerations: Used in PBC too

4.7 – RESPIRATORY MEDICATIONS (EXTENDED LIST)

BRONCHODILATORS – BETA-2 AGONISTS

- Albuterol (ProAir, Ventolin)

Indications: Acute bronchospasm, asthma

Dose: 90 mcg/inhalation, 2 puffs q4–6h PRN

Side Effects: Tachycardia, tremor

Nursing Considerations: Use before steroid inhalers

- Levalbuterol (Xopenex)

Indications: Bronchospasm

Dose: 45 mcg/puff, 2 puffs q4–6h PRN

Side Effects: Less tachycardia than albuterol

Nursing Considerations: Used in sensitive patients

- Salmeterol (Serevent)

Indications: Long-term asthma/COPD control

Dose: 1 inhalation BID

Side Effects: Headache, throat irritation

Nursing Considerations: Not for acute attacks

- Formoterol (Foradil)

Indications: Asthma, COPD

Dose: 1 inhalation BID

Side Effects: Nervousness

Nursing Considerations: Use with corticosteroid

- Arformoterol (Brovana)

Indications: COPD maintenance

Dose: 15 mcg BID via nebulizer

Side Effects: Tremor, QT prolongation

Nursing Considerations: For long-term use only

INHALED CORTICOSTEROIDS

- Fluticasone (Flovent)

Indications: Asthma, COPD

Dose: 100–500 mcg BID

Side Effects: Oral thrush, hoarseness

Nursing Considerations: Rinse mouth after use

- Budesonide (Pulmicort)

Indications: Asthma

Dose: 180–360 mcg BID

Side Effects: Cough, sore throat

Nursing Considerations: Use with spacer

- Beclomethasone (Qvar)

Indications: Asthma

Dose: 40–160 mcg BID

Side Effects: Nasal congestion

Nursing Considerations: Maintenance therapy

- Mometasone (Asmanex)

Indications: Asthma

Dose: 220 mcg once or twice daily

Side Effects: Headache

Nursing Considerations: Not for acute relief

- Ciclesonide (Alvesco)

Indications: Asthma

Dose: 80–160 mcg/day

Side Effects: Throat irritation

Nursing Considerations: Activate before first use

COMBINATION ICS + LABA

- Fluticasone/Salmeterol (Advair)

Indications: Asthma, COPD

Dose: 1 puff BID

Side Effects: Oral thrush, headache

Nursing Considerations: Rinse mouth after use

- Budesonide/Formoterol (Symbicort)

Indications: Asthma, COPD

Dose: 2 puffs BID

Side Effects: Tachycardia, cough

Nursing Considerations: Do not use more than prescribed

- Mometasone/Formoterol (Dulera)

Indications: Asthma

Dose: 2 puffs BID

Side Effects: Dry mouth

Nursing Considerations: Monitor symptom control

- Fluticasone/Vilanterol (Breo Ellipta)

Indications: COPD, asthma

Dose: 1 puff daily

Side Effects: Throat irritation

Nursing Considerations: Once-daily use

ANTICHOLINERGICS
- Ipratropium (Atrovent)

Indications: COPD, asthma adjunct

Dose: 2 puffs QID

Side Effects: Dry mouth, bitter taste

Nursing Considerations: Used with albuterol

- Tiotropium (Spiriva)

Indications: COPD maintenance

Dose: 1 capsule via HandiHaler daily

Side Effects: Throat irritation

Nursing Considerations: Not for acute relief

- Aclidinium (Tudorza)

Indications: COPD

Dose: 400 mcg BID

Side Effects: Headache

Nursing Considerations: Dry powder inhaler

- Glycopyrrolate (Seebri Neohaler)

Indications: COPD

Dose: 15.6 mcg BID

Side Effects: Dry mouth

Nursing Considerations: Not for asthma

- Umeclidinium (Incruse Ellipta)

Indications: COPD

Dose: 62.5 mcg once daily

Side Effects: Cough, sore throat

Nursing Considerations: Inhaled LAMA

MUCOLYTICS AND EXPECTORANTS

- Guaifenesin (Mucinex)

Indications: Productive cough

Dose: 200–400 mg q4h (max 2400 mg/day)

Side Effects: Nausea

Nursing Considerations: Increase fluid intake

- Acetylcysteine (Mucomyst)

Indications: Thick secretions, acetaminophen overdose

Dose: Nebulizer or PO/IV

Side Effects: Bronchospasm

Nursing Considerations: Unpleasant odor

- Dornase alfa (Pulmozyme)

Indications: Cystic fibrosis

Dose: 2.5 mg inhaled daily

Side Effects: Voice alteration

Nursing Considerations: Refrigerate solution

ANTIHISTAMINES – H1 BLOCKERS

- Diphenhydramine (Benadryl)

Indications: Allergies, anaphylaxis adjunct

Dose: 25–50 mg q4–6h

Side Effects: Drowsiness, dry mouth

Nursing Considerations: Avoid driving

- Loratadine (Claritin)

Indications: Allergic rhinitis

Dose: 10 mg/day

Side Effects: Headache

Nursing Considerations: Non-sedating

- Cetirizine (Zyrtec)

Indications: Allergies

Dose: 5–10 mg/day

Side Effects: Fatigue

Nursing Considerations: Monitor for drowsiness

- Fexofenadine (Allegra)

Indications: Seasonal allergies

Dose: 60–180 mg/day

Side Effects: Headache

Nursing Considerations: Take with water

- Levocetirizine (Xyzal)

Indications: Allergic symptoms

Dose: 5 mg at bedtime

Side Effects: Sleepiness

Nursing Considerations: Monitor renal function

LEUKOTRIENE RECEPTOR ANTAGONISTS
- Montelukast (Singulair)

Indications: Asthma, allergies

Dose: 10 mg at bedtime

Side Effects: Mood changes, headache

Nursing Considerations: Not for acute attacks

- Zafirlukast (Accolate)

Indications: Asthma

Dose: 20 mg BID

Side Effects: Liver dysfunction

Nursing Considerations: Take on empty stomach

OTHER RESPIRATORY AGENTS
- Omalizumab (Xolair)

Indications: Severe allergic asthma

Dose: 150–375 mg SQ q2–4 weeks

Side Effects: Injection site reaction

Nursing Considerations: Monitor for anaphylaxis

- Theophylline

Indications: Asthma, COPD

Dose: 200–600 mg/day

Side Effects: Toxicity: nausea, arrhythmia

Nursing Considerations: Monitor serum levels

- Roflumilast (Daliresp)

Indications: Severe COPD

Dose: 500 mcg/day

Side Effects: Weight loss, insomnia

Nursing Considerations: Not a bronchodilator

- Epinephrine (Adrenalin)

Indications: Anaphylaxis, severe asthma

Dose: 0.3–0.5 mg IM

Side Effects: Tachycardia, anxiety

Nursing Considerations: Auto-injector form

- Phenylephrine (Neo-Synephrine)

Indications: Nasal congestion

Dose: 1 spray/nostril q4h PRN

Side Effects: Rebound congestion

Nursing Considerations: Short-term use

4.8 – IMMUNE SYSTEM MEDICATIONS (EXTENDED LIST)

VACCINES
- Influenza vaccine

Indications: Prevention of influenza

Dose: 0.5 mL IM annually

Side Effects: Injection site soreness, mild fever

Nursing Considerations: Assess for egg allergy

- COVID-19 mRNA vaccines (Pfizer, Moderna)

Indications: COVID-19 prevention

Dose: 0.3–0.5 mL IM in 2–3 dose series

Side Effects: Myalgia, fever

Nursing Considerations: Observe 15 min after injection

- Hepatitis B vaccine

Indications: Hepatitis B prevention

Dose: 3 dose series: 0, 1, 6 months

Side Effects: Injection site pain

Nursing Considerations: Check titers in healthcare workers

- MMR (Measles, Mumps, Rubella)

Indications: Childhood immunization

Dose: 0.5 mL SQ at 12 months, then 4–6 yrs

Side Effects: Fever, rash

Nursing Considerations: Live vaccine

- Varicella (Varivax)

Indications: Chickenpox prevention

Dose: 0.5 mL SQ x2 doses

Side Effects: Soreness, mild rash

Nursing Considerations: Live vaccine, avoid in pregnancy

- Tdap (Adacel, Boostrix)

Indications: Tetanus, diphtheria, pertussis

Dose: 0.5 mL IM every 10 years

Side Effects: Pain, low-grade fever

Nursing Considerations: Boost in pregnancy

- HPV vaccine (Gardasil 9)

Indications: HPV prevention

Dose: 0.5 mL IM in 2 or 3 doses

Side Effects: Syncope, pain

Nursing Considerations: Start at age 11–12

- Meningococcal vaccine

Indications: Meningitis prevention

Dose: 0.5 mL IM at 11–12 and 16 yrs

Side Effects: Headache, fatigue

Nursing Considerations: Required for college students

- Pneumococcal vaccine (PPSV23, PCV13)

Indications: Pneumonia prevention

Dose: 0.5 mL IM once or in series

Side Effects: Arm soreness

Nursing Considerations: Indicated in elderly and high-risk

IMMUNOGLOBULINS
- Rho(D) immune globulin (RhoGAM)

Indications: Prevention of Rh sensitization

Dose: 300 mcg IM at 28 weeks & postpartum

Side Effects: Mild fever, site pain

Nursing Considerations: Verify Rh status and Coombs test

- Hepatitis B immune globulin (HBIG)

Indications: Post-exposure prophylaxis

Dose: 0.06 mL/kg IM

Side Effects: Injection site pain

Nursing Considerations: Administer with vaccine for exposure

- Tetanus immune globulin

Indications: Wound management

Dose: 250–500 units IM

Side Effects: Mild reactions

Nursing Considerations: Administer with Td vaccine

- Varicella-Zoster immune globulin (VZIG)

Indications: Varicella exposure in high risk

Dose: Weight-based IM/IV

Side Effects: Mild reactions

Nursing Considerations: Use within 96 hours of exposure

IMMUNOSUPPRESSANTS – TRANSPLANT & AUTOIMMUNE

- Cyclosporine (Neoral, Sandimmune)

Indications: Organ transplant, autoimmune

Dose: 2–12 mg/kg/day

Side Effects: Nephrotoxicity, hirsutism

Nursing Considerations: Monitor trough levels and renal function

- Tacrolimus (Prograf)

Indications: Transplant rejection prevention

Dose: 0.1–0.2 mg/kg/day

Side Effects: Neurotoxicity, hyperglycemia

Nursing Considerations: Monitor drug levels, BP, glucose

- Mycophenolate mofetil (CellCept)

Indications: Transplant, lupus

Dose: 1–3 g/day in divided doses

Side Effects: GI upset, leukopenia

Nursing Considerations: Take on empty stomach

- Azathioprine (Imuran)

Indications: Transplant, RA

Dose: 1–3 mg/kg/day

Side Effects: Bone marrow suppression

Nursing Considerations: Check CBC, LFTs regularly

- Sirolimus (Rapamune)

Indications: Renal transplant

Dose: 2–5 mg/day

Side Effects: Hyperlipidemia, thrombocytopenia

Nursing Considerations: Avoid grapefruit juice

BIOLOGIC AGENTS – AUTOIMMUNE/INFLAMMATORY

- Adalimumab (Humira)

Indications: RA, Crohn's, psoriasis

Dose: 40 mg SQ every other week

Side Effects: Injection site reactions, infections

Nursing Considerations: Screen for TB before start

- Etanercept (Enbrel)

Indications: RA, psoriasis

Dose: 50 mg SQ weekly

Side Effects: Infection risk

Nursing Considerations: Refrigerate, rotate sites

- Infliximab (Remicade)

Indications: RA, Crohn's

Dose: IV infusion q6–8 weeks

Side Effects: Infusion reaction

Nursing Considerations: Premedicate if needed

- Rituximab (Rituxan)

Indications: RA, lymphoma

Dose: IV infusion

Side Effects: Infusion reaction, neutropenia

Nursing Considerations: Screen for hepatitis B

- Tocilizumab (Actemra)

Indications: RA

Dose: IV or SQ dosing

Side Effects: Increased cholesterol, liver enzymes

Nursing Considerations: Monitor labs during treatment

4.9 – RENAL AND URINARY MEDICATIONS (EXTENDED LIST)

DIURETICS

- Furosemide (Lasix)

Indications: Edema, CHF, hypertension

Dose: 20–80 mg/day or more

Side Effects: Hypokalemia, dehydration

Nursing Considerations: Monitor electrolytes, daily weight

- Hydrochlorothiazide (HCTZ)

Indications: Hypertension, mild edema

Dose: 12.5–50 mg/day

Side Effects: Hypokalemia, hyperglycemia

Nursing Considerations: Monitor BP, K+

- Bumetanide (Bumex)

Indications: CHF, edema

Dose: 0.5–2 mg/day

Side Effects: Electrolyte loss

Nursing Considerations: Stronger than furosemide

- Chlorthalidone

Indications: Hypertension

Dose: 12.5–25 mg/day

Side Effects: Photosensitivity, low K+

Nursing Considerations: Preferred thiazide for HTN

- Torsemide (Demadex)

Indications: CHF, hypertension

Dose: 5–20 mg/day

Side Effects: Hypokalemia

Nursing Considerations: Longer duration of action

- Metolazone (Zaroxolyn)

Indications: CHF, resistant edema

Dose: 2.5–10 mg/day

Side Effects: Severe diuresis

Nursing Considerations: Use with loop diuretic

- Spironolactone (Aldactone)

Indications: HF, ascites, PCOS

Dose: 25–100 mg/day

Side Effects: Hyperkalemia, gynecomastia

Nursing Considerations: Avoid in renal failure

- Eplerenone (Inspra)

Indications: Heart failure, HTN

Dose: 25–50 mg/day

Side Effects: Less endocrine effects

Nursing Considerations: Monitor K+, creatinine

- Amiloride

Indications: Hypertension, CHF

Dose: 5–10 mg/day

Side Effects: Hyperkalemia

Nursing Considerations: K+-sparing effect

- Triamterene/HCTZ (Maxzide)

Indications: HTN, fluid retention

Dose: 37.5/25 mg daily

Side Effects: Hyperkalemia, photosensitivity

Nursing Considerations: Combination product

URINARY ANTISPASMODICS

- Oxybutynin (Ditropan)

Indications: Overactive bladder

Dose: 5–15 mg/day or patch

Side Effects: Dry mouth, constipation

Nursing Considerations: Monitor for urinary retention

- Tolterodine (Detrol)

Indications: Urinary incontinence

Dose: 2–4 mg/day

Side Effects: Dizziness, dry eyes

Nursing Considerations: Extended release available

- Solifenacin (Vesicare)

Indications: OAB symptoms

Dose: 5–10 mg/day

Side Effects: QT prolongation

Nursing Considerations: Use with caution in elderly

- Darifenacin (Enablex)

Indications: Urinary urgency

Dose: 7.5–15 mg/day

Side Effects: Dry mouth

Nursing Considerations: May worsen glaucoma

- Mirabegron (Myrbetriq)

Indications: OAB

Dose: 25–50 mg/day

Side Effects: Increased BP

Nursing Considerations: Beta-3 agonist

MEDICATIONS FOR URINARY TRACT INFECTIONS

- Nitrofurantoin (Macrobid)

Indications: Uncomplicated UTI

Dose: 100 mg BID x5–7 days

Side Effects: GI upset, brown urine

Nursing Considerations: Avoid if CrCl <60 mL/min

- Trimethoprim-sulfamethoxazole (Bactrim)

Indications: UTI, pyelonephritis

Dose: 800/160 mg BID

Side Effects: Rash, hyperkalemia

Nursing Considerations: Check for sulfa allergy

- Fosfomycin (Monurol)

Indications: Uncomplicated UTI

Dose: 3 g PO single dose

Side Effects: Diarrhea

Nursing Considerations: Dissolve powder in water

- Ciprofloxacin (Cipro)

Indications: Complicated UTI

Dose: 250–500 mg BID

Side Effects: Tendon rupture risk

Nursing Considerations: Avoid in pregnancy

- Phenazopyridine (Pyridium)

Indications: Urinary tract pain relief

Dose: 100–200 mg TID

Side Effects: Orange/red urine

Nursing Considerations: Short-term use only

PHOSPHATE BINDERS (FOR CKD/ESRD)

- Sevelamer (Renvela)

Indications: Hyperphosphatemia

Dose: 800–1600 mg TID with meals

Side Effects: Nausea, constipation

Nursing Considerations: Non-calcium binder

- Calcium acetate (PhosLo)

Indications: CKD-related hyperphosphatemia

Dose: 667–1334 mg TID with meals

Side Effects: Hypercalcemia

Nursing Considerations: Check calcium/phosphate

- Lanthanum carbonate (Fosrenol)

Indications: Hyperphosphatemia in ESRD

Dose: 500–1500 mg TID

Side Effects: GI distress

Nursing Considerations: Chew tablet before swallowing

ERYTHROPOIESIS-STIMULATING AGENTS

- Epoetin alfa (Epogen, Procrit)

Indications: Anemia due to CKD

Dose: 50–100 units/kg 3x/week

Side Effects: HTN, clot risk

Nursing Considerations: Monitor Hgb, iron

- Darbepoetin alfa (Aranesp)

Indications: CKD anemia

Dose: 0.45 mcg/kg weekly or biweekly

Side Effects: HTN

Nursing Considerations: Do not overcorrect Hgb quickly

OTHER RENAL MEDICATIONS

- Sodium polystyrene sulfonate (Kayexalate)

Indications: Hyperkalemia

Dose: 15–60 g orally or rectally

Side Effects: Diarrhea, hypocalcemia

Nursing Considerations: Monitor K+ closely

- Patiromer (Veltassa)

Indications: Chronic hyperkalemia

Dose: 8.4–25.2 g/day

Side Effects: Constipation

Nursing Considerations: Separate from other meds by 3 hrs

- Calcium carbonate

Indications: Phosphate binder, calcium supplement

Dose: 500–1000 mg with meals

Side Effects: Constipation

Nursing Considerations: Monitor serum calcium

- Cinacalcet (Sensipar)

Indications: Secondary hyperparathyroidism

Dose: 30–180 mg/day

Side Effects: Hypocalcemia

Nursing Considerations: Take with food

4.10 – WOMEN'S AND MEN'S HEALTH MEDICATIONS (EXTENDED LIST)

ORAL CONTRACEPTIVES AND HORMONAL CONTRACEPTION

- Ethinyl estradiol/norgestimate (Ortho Tri-Cyclen)

Indications: Contraception, acne

Dose: 1 tablet daily

Side Effects: Nausea, clot risk

Nursing Considerations: Take at same time daily

- Ethinyl estradiol/levonorgestrel (Seasonique)

Indications: Contraception (extended cycle)

Dose: 1 tablet daily

Side Effects: Breakthrough bleeding

Nursing Considerations: Only 4 periods/year

- Drospirenone/ethinyl estradiol (Yaz)

Indications: PMDD, contraception

Dose: 1 tablet daily

Side Effects: Hyperkalemia

Nursing Considerations: Avoid with renal impairment

- Norethindrone (Micronor)

Indications: Progestin-only contraception

Dose: 1 tablet daily

Side Effects: Irregular bleeding

Nursing Considerations: Must take at same time daily

- Levonorgestrel (Plan B One-Step)

Indications: Emergency contraception

Dose: 1.5 mg single dose

Side Effects: Nausea, menstrual changes

Nursing Considerations: Use within 72 hrs

- Medroxyprogesterone (Depo-Provera)

Indications: Contraception

Dose: 150 mg IM every 3 months

Side Effects: Weight gain, amenorrhea

Nursing Considerations: Delay in return to fertility

- Etonogestrel/ethinyl estradiol (NuvaRing)

Indications: Contraception

Dose: Insert vaginal ring for 3 weeks

Side Effects: Vaginal irritation

Nursing Considerations: Refrigerate before use

- Etonogestrel implant (Nexplanon)

Indications: Long-term contraception

Dose: Subdermal implant x3 years

Side Effects: Irregular bleeding

Nursing Considerations: Requires insertion/removal

- Levonorgestrel IUD (Mirena)

Indications: Contraception, heavy menses

Dose: Intrauterine 3–8 years

Side Effects: Pelvic pain, expulsion

Nursing Considerations: Requires provider placement

HORMONE REPLACEMENT THERAPY

- Conjugated estrogens (Premarin)

Indications: Menopausal symptoms

Dose: 0.3–1.25 mg/day

Side Effects: Breast tenderness, VTE

Nursing Considerations: Lowest effective dose

- Estradiol patch (Vivelle-Dot)

Indications: Menopause

Dose: 0.025–0.1 mg/day patch

Side Effects: Skin irritation

Nursing Considerations: Change site twice weekly

- Estradiol/medroxyprogesterone (Prempro)

Indications: Postmenopausal HRT

Dose: 1 tablet daily

Side Effects: CV risk

Nursing Considerations: Use in women with uterus

- Progesterone (Prometrium)

Indications: Endometrial protection

Dose: 100–200 mg daily

Side Effects: Drowsiness

Nursing Considerations: Take at bedtime

FERTILITY AGENTS
- Clomiphene (Clomid)

Indications: Ovulation induction

Dose: 50–100 mg/day x5 days

Side Effects: Multiple births, hot flashes

Nursing Considerations: Monitor ovulation response

- Letrozole (Femara)

Indications: Ovulation induction, breast cancer

Dose: 2.5–5 mg/day

Side Effects: Fatigue, dizziness

Nursing Considerations: Off-label fertility use

- Menotropins (Menopur)

Indications: Stimulate follicle growth

Dose: IM/SQ dosing per protocol

Side Effects: Ovarian hyperstimulation

Nursing Considerations: Used with hCG

- hCG (Pregnyl, Novarel)

Indications: Trigger ovulation

Dose: 5,000–10,000 IU IM

Side Effects: Abdominal pain

Nursing Considerations: Used after FSH agents

UROGENITAL AND SEXUAL HEALTH (WOMEN)
- Fluconazole (Diflucan)

Indications: Vaginal candidiasis

Dose: 150 mg single dose

Side Effects: GI upset

Nursing Considerations: Avoid in pregnancy

- Metronidazole (Flagyl)

Indications: BV, trichomoniasis

Dose: 500 mg BID x7 days

Side Effects: Metallic taste, no alcohol

Nursing Considerations: Complete full course

- Ospemifene (Osphena)

Indications: Dyspareunia (menopause)

Dose: 60 mg/day

Side Effects: Hot flashes, VTE risk

Nursing Considerations: Take with food

- Estradiol vaginal cream (Estrace)

Indications: Vaginal atrophy

Dose: Apply nightly x2 wks, then 1–3x/week

Side Effects: Local irritation

Nursing Considerations: Counsel on application

ERECTILE DYSFUNCTION (MEN)
- Sildenafil (Viagra)

Indications: ED

Dose: 25–100 mg 1 hr before activity

Side Effects: Flushing, headache

Nursing Considerations: Avoid nitrates

- Tadalafil (Cialis)

Indications: ED, BPH

Dose: 10–20 mg PRN or 2.5–5 mg daily

Side Effects: Back pain, myalgia

Nursing Considerations: Longer half-life

- Vardenafil (Levitra)

Indications: ED

Dose: 5–20 mg 1 hr before sex

Side Effects: Nasal congestion

Nursing Considerations: Avoid high-fat meals

- Avanafil (Stendra)

Indications: ED

Dose: 50–200 mg 30 min before sex

Side Effects: Visual disturbances

Nursing Considerations: Faster onset

BENIGN PROSTATIC HYPERPLASIA (BPH)
- Tamsulosin (Flomax)

Indications: BPH

Dose: 0.4 mg daily

Side Effects: Dizziness, retrograde ejaculation

Nursing Considerations: Take 30 min after same meal

- Alfuzosin (Uroxatral)

Indications: BPH

Dose: 10 mg daily

Side Effects: Hypotension

Nursing Considerations: Extended-release tablet

- Doxazosin (Cardura)

Indications: BPH, HTN

Dose: 1–8 mg/day

Side Effects: Orthostatic hypotension

Nursing Considerations: Give at bedtime

- Finasteride (Proscar)

Indications: BPH, hair loss

Dose: 5 mg/day

Side Effects: Decreased libido

Nursing Considerations: Pregnant women avoid handling

- Dutasteride (Avodart)

Indications: BPH

Dose: 0.5 mg/day

Side Effects: Impotence

Nursing Considerations: Takes months to work

TESTOSTERONE REPLACEMENT (MEN)

- Testosterone gel (AndroGel)

Indications: Hypogonadism

Dose: Apply to shoulders/arms daily

Side Effects: Skin irritation, acne

Nursing Considerations: Wash hands after applying

- Testosterone cypionate (Depo-Testosterone)

Indications: Low testosterone

Dose: IM every 1–4 weeks

Side Effects: Mood swings

Nursing Considerations: Monitor PSA, Hgb

- Testosterone patch (Androderm)

Indications: Hypogonadism

Dose: 4 mg nightly

Side Effects: Irritation, insomnia

Nursing Considerations: Rotate sites

5. ADVERSE EFFECTS & DRUG INTERACTIONS

5.1 RECOGNIZING ADVERSE DRUG REACTIONS (ADRS)

Adverse Drug Reactions (ADRs) are unintended, harmful responses to a medication administered at normal doses for prophylaxis, diagnosis, or therapy. Recognizing ADRs early is a **critical responsibility of the nurse**, as many adverse reactions can escalate rapidly, compromise patient safety, and lead to hospitalization or death if unaddressed.

This section outlines the types of ADRs, clinical warning signs, patient risk factors, and how nurses can act promptly and appropriately in clinical settings.

TYPES OF ADVERSE DRUG REACTIONS

ADRs are typically classified into the following categories:

- **Type A (Augmented):** Dose-dependent, predictable reactions based on pharmacologic properties.
  EXAMPLE: HYPOTENSION FROM ANTIHYPERTENSIVES.
- **Type B (Bizarre):** Unpredictable, not dose-related; often immunologic or idiosyncratic.
  EXAMPLE: ANAPHYLAXIS AFTER A SINGLE PENICILLIN DOSE.

- **Type C (Chronic):** Occur after prolonged therapy.
  EXAMPLE: ADRENAL SUPPRESSION WITH LONG-TERM CORTICOSTEROID USE.
- **Type D (Delayed):** Emerge after drug exposure has ended.
  EXAMPLE: CANCER YEARS AFTER CHEMOTHERAPY.
- **Type E (End-of-use):** Related to drug withdrawal.
  EXAMPLE: BENZODIAZEPINE WITHDRAWAL SEIZURES.
- **Type F (Failure):** Drug fails to produce intended therapeutic effect.
  EXAMPLE: ANTIBIOTIC RESISTANCE LEADING TO INFECTION PROGRESSION.

COMMON SIGNS AND SYMPTOMS OF ADRS

SYSTEMIC INDICATORS TO MONITOR

System	Common Reactions
Skin	Rash, urticaria, pruritus, flushing, blistering
Respiratory	Dyspnea, wheezing, bronchospasm, stridor
Cardiovascular	Hypotension, tachycardia, arrhythmias
GI	Nausea, vomiting, diarrhea, abdominal pain
Neuro	Dizziness, confusion, agitation, seizures
Renal/Hepatic	Jaundice, dark urine, elevated BUN/creatinine

System	Common Reactions
Hematologic	Bleeding, bruising, thrombocytopenia, anemia

HIGH-RISK DRUG CLASSES FOR ADRS

- **Antibiotics:** Allergic reactions, nephrotoxicity
- **NSAIDs:** GI bleeding, renal impairment
- **Opioids:** Respiratory depression, sedation
- **Chemotherapy agents:** Bone marrow suppression, mucositis
- **Antipsychotics:** Neuroleptic malignant syndrome, extrapyramidal symptoms
- **Anticoagulants:** Major bleeding, hematoma formation

PATIENT RISK FACTORS FOR ADRS

- Age extremes (neonates and older adults)
- Polypharmacy and drug interactions
- Renal or hepatic impairment
- History of allergies or hypersensitivity
- Genetic factors (e.g., enzyme polymorphisms)
- Comorbidities that alter drug metabolism or excretion

NURSING ROLE IN RECOGNIZING ADRS

1. **Assessment**

- Perform thorough baseline and ongoing assessments (vitals, physical status, mental status).
- Review lab results and trends (CBC, LFTs, renal panel, coagulation studies).

2. **Monitoring**
   - Monitor closely after initiating new medications or adjusting dosages.
   - Be alert for early, subtle changes in condition.
3. **Documentation**
   - Record onset, duration, and severity of symptoms.
   - Note medication name, route, dose, and timing relative to reaction.
4. **Communication**
   - Report suspected ADRs to the healthcare provider immediately.
   - Notify the pharmacy if necessary.
   - Use institutional reporting tools or national databases (e.g., FDA MedWatch).
5. **Patient Advocacy**
   - Support discontinuation or substitution of the medication if warranted.
   - Educate the patient on ADR symptoms and when to seek help.
   - Ensure allergy and reaction information is clearly documented in the chart.

5.2 REPORTING & MANAGING REACTIONS

Recognizing an adverse drug reaction (ADR) is only the first step. Prompt and effective **reporting and management** of ADRs are essential to ensure patient safety, prevent recurrence, and contribute to improved pharmacovigilance. Nurses serve as front-line reporters and responders in this process.

This section outlines the procedures and best practices for evaluating, documenting, escalating, and managing ADRs in various clinical settings.

IMMEDIATE RESPONSE TO SUSPECTED ADRS

When an ADR is suspected:

1. **Stop the medication** (unless life-sustaining and ordered to continue).
2. **Assess and stabilize** the patient—airway, breathing, circulation (ABCs).
3. **Notify the provider** immediately with concise, accurate clinical information.
4. **Document the event clearly** and in real time.
5. **Monitor for progression or complications**, especially in moderate-to-severe reactions.

MANAGING MILD TO MODERATE ADRS

Examples include nausea, mild rash, dizziness, or headache.

Nursing Interventions:

- Provide supportive care (e.g., antiemetics, fluids, rest).
- Continue monitoring for worsening signs.
- Educate the patient about the reaction and symptom relief.
- Notify the prescriber to evaluate need for dosage adjustment or substitution.

MANAGING SEVERE OR LIFE-THREATENING ADRS

Examples include anaphylaxis, angioedema, respiratory depression, severe hypotension, or organ failure.

Nursing Actions:

- Administer emergency medications as ordered (e.g., epinephrine, diphenhydramine, corticosteroids, naloxone).
- Activate the **Rapid Response Team** or **Code Blue** if necessary.
- Maintain IV access and administer fluids or oxygen support.
- Remain with the patient and continuously assess vital signs and mental status.

REPORTING ADVERSE DRUG REACTIONS

Accurate and timely reporting helps identify patterns of harm, informs regulatory actions, and improves future prescribing practices.

INSTITUTIONAL REPORTING

- Complete the facility's internal **incident or adverse event form**.
- Include full details: drug name, dose, route, time, reaction characteristics, interventions taken, and outcome.
- Submit through risk management or designated safety systems.

NATIONAL REPORTING SYSTEMS

- **FDA MedWatch:**
  Nurses, patients, and providers can report ADRs directly to the FDA via www.fda.gov/medwatch.
- **ISMP (Institute for Safe Medication Practices):**
  Accepts confidential reports on errors and ADRs to inform safety alerts and publications.

DOCUMENTATION BEST PRACTICES

- Be objective, clear, and detailed.
- Include patient statements (e.g., "I feel dizzy," "My throat is swelling").
- Do not assign blame—focus on facts and clinical observations.

FOLLOW-UP CARE AND PATIENT EDUCATION

- Reassess the patient at regular intervals.
- Adjust the plan of care as needed based on recovery or new symptoms.
- Ensure **allergies and adverse reactions** are updated in the health record and clearly flagged.
- Educate the patient and family about the reaction, implications for future medication use, and how to communicate it to other healthcare providers.

THE NURSE'S ROLE IN PREVENTING RECURRENCE

- Identify possible **drug-drug interactions** or underlying risk factors that may have contributed.
- Collaborate with the care team to find safer alternatives.
- Participate in **team debriefings** or root cause analysis (RCA) if the reaction caused harm or required resuscitative efforts.
- Promote a **non-punitive safety culture** by reporting all suspected ADRs, including near-misses.

5.3 COMMON DRUG-DRUG & DRUG-FOOD INTERACTIONS

Drug interactions occur when the effects of one medication are altered by the presence of another substance—**either another drug or a type of food**. These interactions may lead to reduced effectiveness, increased toxicity, or unexpected side effects.

Nurses play a critical role in identifying potential interactions during medication reconciliation, patient education, and ongoing monitoring. Understanding **high-risk combinations** is essential to prevent harm and ensure safe pharmacologic care.

TYPES OF INTERACTIONS

1. DRUG-DRUG INTERACTIONS (DDIS)

Occur when two or more medications interfere with each other's absorption, metabolism, distribution, or excretion.

Types:

- **Additive or synergistic effects** (e.g., two CNS depressants increasing sedation)
- **Antagonistic effects** (e.g., one drug reduces the effect of another)
- **Altered metabolism** via cytochrome P450 enzyme system
- **Competition for protein binding sites**, leading to increased free drug levels

2. DRUG-FOOD INTERACTIONS

Result from specific nutrients or substances in food altering drug absorption, metabolism, or action.

Types:

- Reduced absorption (e.g., calcium binding certain antibiotics)
- Enzyme inhibition or activation
- Altered gastric pH or motility

COMMON DRUG-DRUG INTERACTIONS

Drug 1	Drug 2	Interaction	Nursing Consideration
Warfarin	NSAIDs	Increased bleeding risk	Monitor INR; avoid combo if possible
ACE inhibitors	Potassium-sparing diuretics	Risk of hyperkalemia	Monitor serum potassium
Opioids	Benzodiazepines	Respiratory depression	Avoid combination unless closely monitored
Digoxin	Loop diuretics	Risk of digoxin toxicity (low K+)	Monitor electrolytes and digoxin levels
SSRIs	Triptans or MAOIs	Serotonin syndrome	Observe for confusion, fever, agitation
Macrolide	Statins	Increased statin levels	Consider alternative

Drug 1	Drug 2	Interaction	Nursing Consideration
antibiotics		(rhabdomyolysis risk)	antibiotic
Fluoroquinolones	Antacids	Reduced antibiotic absorption	Separate administration by at least 2 hours

COMMON DRUG-FOOD INTERACTIONS

Drug	Food	Interaction	Nursing Consideration
Warfarin	Vitamin K-rich foods (e.g., spinach, kale)	Antagonizes effect	Keep intake consistent; monitor INR
MAO inhibitors	Tyramine-rich foods (aged cheese, wine)	Hypertensive crisis	Avoid aged, fermented, pickled foods
Grapefruit juice	Calcium channel blockers, statins	Inhibits CYP3A4 metabolism	Avoid juice; may increase drug levels
Tetracyclines	Milk/dairy (calcium)	Reduced absorption	Take on empty stomach or separate by 2 hours

Drug	Food	Interaction	Nursing Consideration
Levodopa	High-protein meals	Competes with amino acids for absorption	Take on empty stomach or low-protein meal
Iron supplements	Coffee, tea	Reduced absorption	Avoid concurrent intake; take with Vitamin C

NURSING ASSESSMENT AND INTERVENTION STRATEGIES

1. **Medication Reconciliation**
   - Review all prescription and OTC drugs, supplements, and herbals during admission and discharge.
2. **Patient Education**
   - Clearly instruct patients on foods or drugs to avoid.
   - Provide printed information or medication schedules if needed.
3. **Lab Monitoring**
   - Watch for signs of altered drug levels (e.g., INR, electrolytes, creatinine).
   - Assess liver and kidney function for patients on multiple medications.
4. **Timing Adjustments**
   - Separate interacting substances by several hours to reduce interaction risk.
   - Time meals appropriately around medications that require fasting or low-fat content.

HIGH-RISK POPULATIONS

- **Older adults** with polypharmacy
- **Patients with renal or hepatic impairment**
- **Critically ill** or those with altered metabolism
- **Patients with narrow therapeutic index drugs** (e.g., warfarin, lithium, digoxin)

6. IV DRUG ADMINISTRATION GUIDELINES

6.1 IV COMPATIBILITY & MIXING CHART

Intravenous (IV) drug administration provides rapid therapeutic effects, but it also carries a high risk of complications if drugs are **incompatible** when mixed or infused together. IV incompatibility can lead to **precipitation, inactivation, or chemical reactions** that may harm the patient or compromise efficacy.

Nurses must be well-informed about **compatibility guidelines, diluents, and mixing techniques**, especially in high-acuity settings such as intensive care, emergency departments, and perioperative units.

TYPES OF IV INCOMPATIBILITY

1. **Physical Incompatibility**
   - Visible changes such as **cloudiness, precipitates, or color change**.
   - Caused by direct chemical interactions between drugs or between a drug and a solution.

2. **Chemical Incompatibility**
   - Degradation of drug potency due to **pH changes**, oxidation, or hydrolysis.
   - Often not visible but results in loss of drug effectiveness.
3. **Therapeutic Incompatibility**
   - When two drugs with opposing effects are administered together (e.g., a vasoconstrictor with a vasodilator), leading to reduced efficacy.

COMMON INCOMPATIBLE IV DRUG COMBINATIONS

Drug A	Drug B	Result	Notes
Furosemide	Midazolam	Precipitation	Use separate IV lines or flush between medications
Ceftriaxone	Calcium-containing solutions	Fatal precipitate	Never mix in neonates; flush line between uses
Phenytoin	Dextrose	Precipitates	Only compatible with normal saline
Amphotericin B	Many other IV drugs	Highly incompatible	Use dedicated line
Sodium bicarbonate	Dopamine	Reduced dopamine stability	Avoid mixing

Drug A	Drug B	Result	Notes
Heparin	Alteplase (tPA)	Neutralization of effects	Administer separately with sufficient flush

ALWAYS REFER TO INSTITUTIONAL COMPATIBILITY DATABASES (E.G., TRISSEL'S™, MICROMEDEX®) BEFORE COMBINING IV MEDICATIONS.

DILUENT COMPATIBILITY OVERVIEW

Drug	Compatible Diluent	Incompatible Diluent	Nursing Tip
Vancomycin	Normal saline (NS), D5W	Ringer's lactate (may precipitate)	Infuse slowly to avoid red man syndrome
Potassium chloride	NS, D5W	Do not mix with calcium	Never IV push; dilute and administer via pump
Lorazepam (Ativan)	D5W	NS (may cause precipitation)	Use microdrip tubing and glass containers if possible
Metronidazole	NS, D5W	Incompatible with many antibiotics	Protect from light
Nitroprusside	D5W	Avoid NS	Wrap IV bag in opaque

Drug	Compatible Diluent	Incompatible Diluent	Nursing Tip
			covering

BEST PRACTICES FOR IV COMPATIBILITY

1. **Check Before You Mix**
   - Use up-to-date compatibility references or institutional software before combining drugs.
   - Assume incompatibility unless verified.
2. **Flush Between Medications**
   - When administering drugs sequentially via the same IV line, flush with compatible solution (usually 10 mL NS) before and after.
3. **Use Separate Lines When Needed**
   - For drugs that are known to be incompatible or in critically ill patients, use **dedicated lumens or IV lines**.
4. **Label Everything**
   - Clearly mark **IV bags and tubing** with drug name, concentration, time, and initials.
   - Document any changes or additions in the MAR.
5. **Prepare in Pharmacy When Possible**
   - For high-risk drugs (e.g., chemo, TPN, high-dose electrolytes), request **pharmacy-compounded solutions**.
6. **Avoid Mixing at the Bedside**
   - Unless specifically trained and authorized, avoid bedside mixing of IV additives.

NURSING ROLE IN IV SAFETY

- Assess IV site regularly for signs of infiltration, phlebitis, or extravasation.
- Monitor patient response during and after drug infusion.
- Report any **unexpected precipitation, color changes, or patient symptoms** immediately.
- Maintain accurate and complete documentation, including batch numbers for high-risk drugs (e.g., TPN, blood products).

6.2 IV PUSH VS DRIP: RATE & SAFETY

Administering medications intravenously requires **precise knowledge of delivery methods and infusion rates**. Two primary IV techniques are used in clinical practice: **IV push (bolus)** and **IV infusion (drip or pump-controlled)**. Each has specific indications, advantages, risks, and safety protocols.

Nurses must be familiar with drug-specific administration rates, dilution requirements, and monitoring responsibilities to **ensure efficacy and avoid complications** such as extravasation, toxicity, or cardiac events.

IV PUSH (IV BOLUS)

DEFINITION:

A method of delivering medication directly into the bloodstream via syringe over a short time, usually **less than 5 minutes**.

ADVANTAGES:

- Rapid onset of action
- Immediate therapeutic effect
- Useful in emergencies (e.g., naloxone, epinephrine)

RISKS:

- Increased risk of adverse reactions if administered too quickly
- Higher potential for dosing errors
- Requires strict attention to rate and compatibility

NURSING GUIDELINES:

- Check institutional protocols for **rate of administration** for each drug (some require 1–2 minutes, others up to 5 minutes)
- Dilute as recommended (e.g., morphine diluted in 5–10 mL NS)
- Administer **slowly and steadily**, watching for flushing, burning, or discomfort
- Use **patent IV access only**
- Always **flush before and after** with at least 10 mL of NS unless contraindicated
- Monitor patient's vitals and level of consciousness closely during and after administration

COMMON IV PUSH MEDICATIONS AND RECOMMENDED RATES

Medication	Recommended Push Rate
Furosemide	20 mg/min
Morphine sulfate	Over 4–5 minutes
Midazolam	Over 2 minutes
Digoxin	Slow IV over 5 minutes

Medication	Recommended Push Rate
Ketorolac	Over at least 15 seconds
Ondansetron	Over 2–5 minutes

ALWAYS VERIFY UPDATED INSTITUTIONAL POLICIES AND REFERENCES.

IV INFUSION (DRIP OR PUMP)

DEFINITION:

Continuous or intermittent infusion of medication in a diluted form over a set period, typically **using a pump or gravity drip**.

ADVANTAGES:

- Controlled rate reduces risk of toxicity
- Suitable for medications requiring slow, steady absorption
- Allows for concurrent fluid replacement or maintenance therapy

RISKS:

- Risk of infusion pump programming errors
- Infiltration or phlebitis at IV site
- Potential for interactions if infusing multiple medications

NURSING GUIDELINES:

- Use **smart infusion pumps** with drug libraries when available

- Verify **infusion rate (mL/hr or mcg/kg/min)** per order
- Check **compatibility** with diluents and co-infused drugs
- Assess IV site and patient response every hour or as per facility protocol
- Document start and stop times, infusion rates, and any side effects observed

COMMON IV INFUSION MEDICATIONS AND TYPICAL PARAMETERS

Medication	Typical Infusion Parameters
Vancomycin	Infuse over at least 60 minutes (1 g)
Potassium chloride	No faster than 10 mEq/hr via peripheral
Dopamine	2–20 mcg/kg/min (titrated by response)
Magnesium sulfate	1–2 g/hr for preeclampsia or hypomagnesemia
Ceftriaxone	Over 30 minutes (standard dose)

WHEN TO CHOOSE IV PUSH VS. IV INFUSION

Criteria	IV Push	IV Infusion

Criteria	IV Push	IV Infusion
Onset needed	Immediate	Gradual
Duration of action	Short	Sustained
Safety margin	Narrow margin = infusion preferred	Safer for high-risk or irritating meds
Monitoring	Requires continuous observation	Allows periodic reassessment
Drug concentration	High in small volume	Diluted in larger volume

SAFETY REMINDERS

- **Never administer medication IV push into a line with incompatible infusions**
- **Know your drug**: dilution, rate, and required monitoring
- **Educate patients**: warn about sensations (e.g., metallic taste, warmth) during push
- **Use pre-programmed pump settings** when possible to reduce programming errors
- **Use appropriate tubing and filters** per drug requirements

6.3 PREVENTING IV SITE COMPLICATIONS

Intravenous (IV) therapy is essential for delivering medications, fluids, and nutrition directly into the bloodstream. However, it also presents risks for **local and systemic complications**, particularly when IV sites are not properly monitored or maintained. Nurses are responsible for **assessing, maintaining, and protecting the integrity of the IV site**, ensuring that complications are detected early and prevented when possible.

This section outlines the most common IV site complications and evidence-based strategies for prevention and intervention.

COMMON IV SITE COMPLICATIONS

Complication	Definition
Infiltration	Non-vesicant fluid leaks into surrounding tissue
Extravasation	Vesicant medication leaks into tissue, causing possible tissue damage
Phlebitis	Inflammation of the vein, often due to mechanical or chemical irritation
Thrombophlebitis	Phlebitis with presence of a blood clot
Infection	Localized or systemic infection from contaminated site or poor technique
Hematoma	Bleeding into the tissue due to vein rupture or failed insertion

Complication	Definition
Air Embolism	Entry of air into the bloodstream, usually during insertion or removal

SIGNS AND SYMPTOMS TO MONITOR

Complication	Key Signs
Infiltration	Cool, pale, swollen site; slowed or stopped infusion
Extravasation	Burning, pain, blistering, necrosis
Phlebitis	Redness, warmth, cord-like vein, tenderness
Infection	Redness, warmth, purulent drainage, fever
Hematoma	Bruising, swelling, tenderness at site
Air embolism	Dyspnea, chest pain, hypotension, cyanosis

PREVENTION STRATEGIES

1. SITE SELECTION AND CATHETER CHOICE

- Use the **smallest gauge** catheter appropriate for therapy.
- Avoid sites near joints, areas of flexion, or previously damaged veins.
- Rotate IV sites per facility protocol (usually every 72–96 hours for peripheral lines).
- Avoid starting IVs on the same side as a **mastectomy, AV fistula, or infection**.

2. ASEPTIC TECHNIQUE

- Perform **hand hygiene** before insertion and every time accessing the line.
- Use **chlorhexidine** or alcohol for site preparation.
- Maintain a **closed system** and change IV tubing per institutional policy.

3. SECUREMENT AND DRESSING

- Stabilize the catheter using sterile, transparent dressings or securement devices.
- Keep site visible for inspection.
- Change dressings if damp, soiled, or compromised.

4. SITE ASSESSMENT

- Assess the IV site **at least every shift** or per protocol.
- Document site condition, patency, and any patient-reported discomfort.
- Evaluate for signs of redness, swelling, leaking, or pain.

5. MEDICATION ADMINISTRATION

- Confirm **compatibility** of IV medications to prevent irritation or precipitation.
- Dilute and administer **vesicant drugs** (e.g., dopamine, chemotherapy agents) via central line if possible.

- Monitor rate of infusion carefully—rapid administration increases risk of irritation.

IF COMPLICATION OCCURS: NURSING ACTIONS

INFILTRATION

- Stop infusion immediately.
- Elevate the limb and apply warm or cold compresses based on policy.
- Document and restart IV in a different vein.

EXTRAVASATION

- Stop infusion and leave catheter in place.
- Notify provider immediately.
- Administer antidote if applicable (e.g., hyaluronidase).
- Apply appropriate compress and monitor for tissue damage.

PHLEBITIS

- Discontinue IV and apply warm compress.
- Document and consider alternate site for IV insertion.
- Assess need for follow-up (e.g., culture, ultrasound).

INFECTION

- Remove catheter and send tip for culture if ordered.
- Notify provider and monitor vital signs.
- Initiate antibiotics if infection is confirmed.

AIR EMBOLISM

- Clamp tubing immediately.
- Place patient in **left lateral Trendelenburg position**.
- Notify provider and administer oxygen.
- Monitor respiratory and cardiovascular status.

DOCUMENTATION ESSENTIALS

- Record insertion date, site, gauge, and number of attempts.
- Note assessment findings each shift and with any changes.
- Document patient education, interventions for complications, and outcomes.

7. HERBAL, OTC & ALTERNATIVE MEDICATIONS

7.1 COMMON SUPPLEMENTS & PATIENT USE

Herbal supplements and over-the-counter (OTC) remedies are widely used by patients in all healthcare settings. Many assume that because these products are "natural," they are inherently safe—yet they can **cause adverse effects, interact with prescription medications**, and complicate treatment plans.

As frontline healthcare providers, **nurses must assess, educate, and monitor** patients who use supplements. This requires a working knowledge of commonly used herbal products, their intended effects, and their clinical risks.

WHY IT MATTERS IN NURSING

- Herbal supplements are **not regulated** like prescription medications.

- Patients may **not disclose** supplement use unless specifically asked.
- Supplements may **interact with anticoagulants, immunosuppressants, psychotropics**, and many other drug classes.
- Some may alter **lab values**, affect **anesthesia**, or **mimic symptoms** of disease.

COMMON HERBAL SUPPLEMENTS AND THEIR CLINICAL RELEVANCE

Supplement	Common Uses	Clinical Concerns
St. John's Wort	Depression, anxiety, sleep	Induces CYP450; reduces effectiveness of oral contraceptives, warfarin, SSRIs
Ginkgo biloba	Memory support, dementia	Increases bleeding risk; interacts with anticoagulants and NSAIDs
Ginseng	Energy, immune function, diabetes	Can cause insomnia, tachycardia; interacts with warfarin, insulin
Garlic	Cardiovascular health, cholesterol	Increases bleeding risk; avoid with anticoagulants
Echinacea	Colds, flu, immune support	May interfere with immunosuppressants; allergy risk in daisy family
Saw Palmetto	Prostate	May mimic hormonal drugs; avoid

Supplement	Common Uses	Clinical Concerns
	enlargement	with finasteride
Kava	Anxiety, relaxation	Hepatotoxicity risk; avoid with CNS depressants
Valerian Root	Sleep aid, anxiety	Sedation risk; avoid with benzodiazepines, alcohol
Turmeric/Curcumin	Inflammation, joint pain	May affect platelet aggregation; caution in bleeding disorders
Black Cohosh	Menopausal symptoms	Hormonal effects; avoid in hormone-sensitive cancers
Melatonin	Sleep regulation	Can interact with anticoagulants, antidiabetics

NURSING ASSESSMENT QUESTIONS

During admission or medication review, ask patients:

- Are you taking any **vitamins, minerals, herbal products, or supplements**?
- Where do you purchase your supplements?
- Why do you take them? Who recommended them?
- Do you take them at the same time as your prescription medications?

- Have you noticed any side effects?

Document all responses clearly in the **medication reconciliation** process.

KEY POPULATIONS AT HIGHER RISK

- **Older adults** (polypharmacy, renal/hepatic decline)
- **Pregnant or lactating women**
- **Patients undergoing surgery**
- **Patients on anticoagulants or psychotropic medications**
- **Oncology or transplant patients** (immunosuppressed)

NURSING EDUCATION PRIORITIES

- Supplements may alter the **absorption, metabolism, or effectiveness** of prescription drugs.
- "Natural" does **not mean safe**—review FDA alerts or reports of adverse effects.
- Advise patients to bring all supplements to appointments for review.
- Encourage open dialogue—patients may not volunteer this information unless asked in a **non-judgmental** manner.
- Teach patients to **stop certain supplements** (e.g., ginkgo, garlic) **before surgery** to reduce bleeding risk.

CLINICAL REMINDERS

- Herbal supplements are not standardized in dose or purity.
- Monitor for unexpected side effects or signs of interaction.

- Encourage patients to use **USP-verified** or pharmacy-reviewed products.
- Report adverse effects to **FDA MedWatch** if suspected.

7.2 KEY INTERACTIONS WITH PRESCRIPTION DRUGS

Herbal supplements and over-the-counter (OTC) products can interact with prescription medications in ways that are **clinically significant and potentially dangerous**. These interactions may alter drug metabolism, increase toxicity, or reduce therapeutic effect—often without the patient's awareness.

Nurses play a vital role in identifying these interactions through **comprehensive assessments, patient education, and collaboration with the healthcare team**. This section highlights the most clinically relevant and commonly encountered interactions between supplements and prescription drugs.

MECHANISMS OF HERBAL–DRUG INTERACTIONS

- **Enzyme induction or inhibition** (especially CYP450 enzymes): Affects drug metabolism.
- **Alteration of absorption** (e.g., by changing GI motility or pH).
- **Competing for protein-binding sites**: Alters free drug levels in plasma.
- **Additive effects** (e.g., enhanced sedation or anticoagulation).
- **Antagonistic effects**: Supplements may block or reverse medication effects.

HIGH-RISK HERBAL–DRUG INTERACTIONS

Herbal Supplement	Prescription Drug Class	Interaction/Effect	Nursing Concern
St. John's Wort	SSRIs, oral contraceptives, warfarin, cyclosporine	Induces CYP3A4 → ↓ drug levels → treatment failure	Avoid in psychiatric, transplant, contraceptive therapy
Ginkgo biloba	Anticoagulants (warfarin, aspirin)	Increases bleeding risk	Monitor for bruising, bleeding
Ginseng	Insulin, warfarin, digoxin	Hypoglycemia, ↓ warfarin effect, ↑ digoxin toxicity	Monitor glucose, INR, digoxin levels
Garlic	Warfarin, antiplatelets	Increased risk of bleeding	Educate patient to avoid excess garlic
Kava	CNS depressants (benzodiazepines, opioids)	Potentiates sedation and respiratory depression	Contraindicated in sedated or respiratory-compromised patients
Valerian	Sedatives, anesthetics	Additive CNS depression	Discontinue before surgery
Black Cohosh	Hormone replacement therapy, tamoxifen	Possible hormonal interference	Avoid in hormone-sensitive

Herbal Supplement	Prescription Drug Class	Interaction/Effect	Nursing Concern
			conditions
Echinacea	Immunosuppressants	May stimulate immune system, reducing drug efficacy	Avoid in transplant recipients
Melatonin	Anticoagulants, antihypertensives	May alter coagulation and blood pressure	Monitor INR and BP
Licorice (natural)	Diuretics, corticosteroids	Hypokalemia, hypertension	Monitor potassium and BP
Turmeric	Anticoagulants, antidiabetics	↑ bleeding, ↓ glucose	Assess bleeding and hypoglycemia risks

PHARMACOKINETIC VS. PHARMACODYNAMIC INTERACTIONS

- **Pharmacokinetic**: Changes how the drug is **absorbed, metabolized, or eliminated**
  EXAMPLE: St. John's Wort induces enzymes → reduces levels of oral contraceptives
- **Pharmacodynamic**: Changes how the drug **acts on the body** (additive or opposing effects)
  EXAMPLE: Valerian + benzodiazepines → excessive sedation

RED FLAGS FOR POTENTIAL INTERACTIONS

- **New or worsening side effects** after starting a supplement
- **Unexplained loss of therapeutic control** (e.g., elevated INR, unstable blood sugar)
- **Poor response to standard doses** of prescribed medications
- **Duplicate effects** from herbal and prescription drugs (e.g., multiple sedatives)

NURSING STRATEGIES TO PREVENT HARM

1. **Ask specifically about supplement use** during medication history.
2. **Cross-check all supplements** against prescribed medications using drug interaction tools.
3. **Educate patients** on high-risk combinations and encourage transparency.
4. **Document all supplements** in the medication list.
5. **Encourage patients to stop unnecessary supplements** before surgery or medication changes.
6. **Monitor labs and clinical outcomes** more closely in patients using multiple therapies.

7.3 COUNSELING PATIENTS ON SAFE USE

Patient counseling is essential when it comes to **herbal, OTC, and alternative medications**. Many patients self-medicate with supplements based on personal beliefs, advertising, or advice from non-medical sources. Nurses have a unique opportunity to guide patients with **accurate, evidence-based information** that supports safe and informed decision-making.

This section provides practical strategies for counseling patients on the **responsible use of non-prescription products**, helping to avoid risks, interactions, and misinformation.

CORE PRINCIPLES OF SAFE USE COUNSELING

1. **Create a Judgment-Free Environment**
   - Many patients are reluctant to disclose their supplement use unless asked in a respectful, non-judgmental manner.
   - Use open-ended questions like:
     "Can you tell me about any vitamins, herbal products, or natural remedies you take regularly?"
2. **Normalize the Topic**
   - Let patients know it's common to use these products and that discussing them helps prevent unsafe combinations.
3. **Avoid Dismissive Language**
   - Rather than saying, "That doesn't work," frame concerns in a clinically balanced way:
     "There's limited research on this supplement, and I'd like to make sure it's safe to use with your medications."

KEY TEACHING POINTS FOR PATIENTS

1. INFORM ALL PROVIDERS

- Patients should tell all healthcare providers—including dentists and pharmacists—about every supplement they take.
- Emphasize that herbal products can affect surgery, anesthesia, lab results, and drug metabolism.

2. BE CAUTIOUS WITH ONLINE PURCHASES

- Many supplements sold online may contain undisclosed ingredients or variable potencies.
- Recommend products that are **USP-verified** or obtained through **reputable pharmacies**.

3. FOLLOW DOSING GUIDELINES

- Natural does not mean safe in large quantities.
- Warn patients not to exceed recommended dosages or combine multiple products with similar ingredients (e.g., multiple sleep aids).

4. WATCH FOR SIDE EFFECTS AND INTERACTIONS

- Teach patients to monitor for new symptoms after starting a supplement.
- Highlight risks with blood thinners, sedatives, immunosuppressants, or hormonal therapies.

5. USE CAUTION DURING PREGNANCY, SURGERY, AND CHRONIC ILLNESS

- Many supplements are not tested for use during pregnancy or lactation.
- Certain herbs increase the risk of bleeding and should be stopped before surgery (e.g., ginkgo, garlic, ginseng).
- Chronic diseases such as **diabetes, hypertension, and cancer** may be worsened by some "natural" therapies.

SPECIAL POPULATIONS TO EDUCATE CLOSELY

- **Elderly patients** (risk of polypharmacy, altered metabolism)
- **Pregnant and breastfeeding women**
- **Patients with chronic liver or kidney disease**

- Patients on anticoagulants, antiepileptics, or antipsychotics

PRACTICAL RESOURCES TO SHARE

- FDA's MedWatch program for reporting supplement side effects: www.fda.gov/medwatch
- NIH Office of Dietary Supplements: ods.od.nih.gov
- Drug-supplement interaction checkers from Micromedex®, Lexicomp®, or Epocrates®

SAMPLE PATIENT ADVICE SCRIPT

"Even though this product is available over the counter, it may affect your prescription medications or cause unexpected side effects. Let's take a closer look at the ingredients together, and we'll talk about what's safe based on your health conditions and medications."

8. SPECIAL POPULATIONS & CLINICAL SCENARIOS

8.1 EMERGENCY & CRITICAL CARE DRUGS

In emergency and critical care settings, nurses must act with speed, precision, and confidence. The pharmacologic agents used in these high-acuity environments are often **high-risk, rapid-acting medications** with narrow therapeutic windows. Errors can have immediate, life-threatening consequences, making it essential for nurses to understand each drug's purpose, mechanism of action, dosing parameters, and required monitoring.

This section reviews key drugs commonly used in **resuscitation, hemodynamic stabilization, advanced cardiac life support (ACLS), and critical interventions.**

CATEGORIES OF EMERGENCY DRUGS

1. **Cardiac Resuscitation and Rhythm Control**
2. **Hemodynamic Support**
3. **Respiratory and Airway Management**
4. **Reversal Agents**
5. **Electrolyte Emergencies**
6. **Sedation and Rapid Sequence Intubation (RSI)**

KEY EMERGENCY & CRITICAL CARE MEDICATIONS

Drug	Indication	Nursing Considerations
Epinephrine	Cardiac arrest (ACLS), anaphylaxis	1 mg IV/IO every 3–5 min in ACLS; monitor for tachycardia, hypertension
Amiodarone	Ventricular fibrillation, pulseless VT	IV push (300 mg, then 150 mg); continuous ECG, bradycardia risk
Atropine	Symptomatic bradycardia	0.5 mg IV every 3–5 min (max 3 mg); monitor HR, BP

Drug	Indication	Nursing Considerations
Adenosine	Paroxysmal supraventricular tachycardia (PSVT)	Rapid IV push followed by flush; may cause brief asystole
Lidocaine	Ventricular arrhythmias	Watch for CNS toxicity; adjust dose in liver dysfunction
Dopamine	Shock, hypotension, bradycardia	Dose-dependent effects (renal vs cardiac); monitor BP, ECG
Norepinephrine	Septic or cardiogenic shock	Titrate via central line; risk of ischemia at high doses
Phenylephrine	Vasopressor for hypotension	Pure alpha agonist; reflex bradycardia possible
Magnesium sulfate	Torsades de pointes, eclampsia	Monitor for hypotension, respiratory depression, deep tendon reflexes
Sodium bicarbonate	Metabolic acidosis, drug overdoses	Use only when clearly indicated; risk of alkalosis, fluid overload
Naloxone (Narcan)	Opioid overdose	Repeat dosing often required; monitor for re-sedation or agitation

Drug	Indication	Nursing Considerations
Flumazenil	Benzodiazepine overdose	Use with caution—may precipitate seizures
Rocuronium / Succinylcholine	Neuromuscular blockade for intubation	Requires sedation and airway support; monitor paralysis
Etomidate	RSI induction agent	Rapid onset; minimal cardiovascular depression
Ketamine	RSI, sedation, pain	Increases BP and HR; monitor for emergence reactions
Dextrose (D50)	Hypoglycemia	Administer via large bore IV; monitor for rebound hypoglycemia
Calcium gluconate / chloride	Hyperkalemia, calcium channel blocker overdose	Give slowly; monitor ECG, vein patency
Albuterol (neb)	Bronchospasm, asthma	May cause tremors, tachycardia; assess breath sounds before/after

NURSING PRIORITIES IN EMERGENCY DRUG ADMINISTRATION

1. **Rapid Assessment and Prioritization**
    - ABCs (Airway, Breathing, Circulation) guide treatment choices.
    - Perform ongoing reassessments every 2–5 minutes during resuscitation or code.
2. **Know Emergency Protocols**
    - Be proficient in **ACLS, PALS, and institutional emergency pathways**.
    - Use **code carts, defibrillators**, and **smart pumps** correctly and confidently.
3. **Medication Preparation**
    - Know **dilution requirements, compatible fluids, and IV push vs infusion** standards.
    - Label all syringes and infusions accurately.
4. **Use Central Lines When Appropriate**
    - For vasopressors and irritants (e.g., norepinephrine), avoid peripheral administration if possible.
    - Monitor central line patency, site condition, and signs of infection or extravasation.
5. **Monitor Closely for Therapeutic Response and Adverse Effects**
    - Continuously assess vital signs, ECG, oxygenation, and neurologic status.
    - Be prepared to titrate or switch drugs as the clinical picture evolves.
6. **Communicate Clearly and Document Accurately**
    - Verbal orders are common in emergencies—**read back** for confirmation.
    - Document exact doses, times, routes, and patient responses.

8.2 PREGNANCY & LACTATION CONSIDERATIONS

Medication use during pregnancy and lactation presents unique challenges. Physiological changes during these stages alter drug pharmacokinetics, and many medications may pose **risks to the fetus or nursing infant**. Nurses play a critical role in **assessing drug safety, educating patients, and advocating for alternatives** when needed.

This section outlines essential principles, FDA risk categories, and key nursing implications when caring for pregnant or breastfeeding patients receiving medication therapy.

PHARMACOKINETIC CHANGES IN PREGNANCY

- **Increased plasma volume and cardiac output**: Dilutes drug concentration.
- **Decreased GI motility**: May delay drug absorption.
- **Increased renal clearance**: May reduce half-life of renally excreted drugs.
- **Altered hepatic enzyme activity**: Can enhance or reduce metabolism of specific drugs.
- **Placental transfer**: Many drugs cross the placenta and may affect fetal development.

DRUG RISK IN PREGNANCY: FDA LABELING SYSTEM

The old FDA pregnancy categories (A, B, C, D, X) have been **phased out** and replaced by the **Pregnancy and Lactation Labeling Rule (PLLR)**, which includes:

1. **Pregnancy (including Labor & Delivery)**
    - Risks based on human and animal data
    - Clinical considerations and dosing guidance
2. **Lactation**

- Potential for drug transfer via breast milk
- Effects on the infant and milk production
3. **Females & Males of Reproductive Potential**
    - Includes contraception needs and fertility effects

NURSES SHOULD REFERENCE THE PLLR SECTIONS IN CURRENT DRUG GUIDES OR THE FDA DATABASE FOR UP-TO-DATE RISK INFORMATION.

COMMON HIGH-RISK DRUGS IN PREGNANCY

Drug/Class	Risk	Nursing Note
ACE inhibitors	Fetal renal damage, oligohydramnios	Contraindicated in 2nd/3rd trimesters
Warfarin	Teratogenic, fetal bleeding	Use heparin as safer alternative
Isotretinoin (Accutane)	Severe birth defects	Absolute contraindication; iPLEDGE program
NSAIDs	Premature ductus arteriosus closure	Avoid in 3rd trimester
Tetracyclines	Tooth discoloration, impaired bone growth	Avoid during pregnancy
Fluoroquinolones	Fetal cartilage damage (animal data)	Use only if no safer option available

Drug/Class	Risk	Nursing Note
Methotrexate	Abortion, teratogenesis	Contraindicated
Lithium	Congenital heart defects	Use with caution; monitor serum levels
Valproic acid	Neural tube defects	Avoid when possible

DRUG SAFETY IN LACTATION

- Most drugs are **excreted in breast milk** to some degree.
- The **infant's age and metabolism** influence risk.
- Drugs with long half-lives, high lipid solubility, or active metabolites may accumulate.

DRUGS TO AVOID OR USE WITH CAUTION DURING LACTATION

Drug/Class	Lactation Concern	Alternative Recommendation
Chloramphenicol	Bone marrow suppression in infants	Avoid
Ergotamines	Suppress milk production	Use safer migraine treatments
Lithium	High milk levels, toxicity in	Monitor closely or avoid

Drug/Class	Lactation Concern	Alternative Recommendation
	infant	
Radioactive isotopes	Radiation exposure risk	Temporarily stop breastfeeding
Codeine, Tramadol	Risk of CNS depression in infants	Use non-opioid pain relief if possible
Fluoroquinolones	Uncertain safety in infants	Use alternatives if available

NURSING RESPONSIBILITIES

1. **Conduct a Complete Drug History**
   - Include OTC, herbal, and vitamin supplements.
   - Assess for teratogenic risk and drug class safety.
2. **Use Trusted Resources**
   - Reference LactMed (NIH), Briggs' DRUGS IN PREGNANCY AND LACTATION, or FDA labeling.
3. **Patient Education**
   - Emphasize the importance of medication adherence for chronic conditions (e.g., epilepsy, diabetes).
   - Warn against self-discontinuation or over-the-counter medication use without provider approval.
   - Explain potential infant exposure and signs of toxicity.
4. **Monitor Mother and Infant**
   - Watch for maternal side effects and fetal well-being.
   - Assess the breastfeeding infant for changes in feeding, sleep, alertness, or development.

5. **Collaborate with Providers**
    - Advocate for the safest therapeutic options.
    - Request dose adjustments or safer alternatives when needed.

8.3 PEDIATRIC DOSING & SAFETY

Pediatric patients are not simply "small adults." Drug absorption, distribution, metabolism, and excretion vary significantly based on **age, weight, organ maturity, and developmental stage**. Medication errors in children can have **severe or fatal consequences**, making precise calculation and monitoring essential.

This section focuses on principles of safe pediatric dosing, high-risk drug categories, and practical nursing strategies for administering medications to neonates, infants, and children.

KEY DIFFERENCES IN PEDIATRIC PHARMACOKINETICS

Pharmacokinetic Phase	Consideration in Children
Absorption	Gastric pH is higher (less acidic) in neonates; affects drug solubility
Distribution	Higher total body water and lower fat content alter drug dispersion
Metabolism	Immature liver enzyme systems affect drug breakdown (especially <1 year)

Pharmacokinetic Phase	Consideration in Children
Excretion	Reduced renal function in neonates delays drug clearance

THESE DIFFERENCES NECESSITATE DOSING ADJUSTMENTS AND CLOSE MONITORING.

PRINCIPLES OF PEDIATRIC DOSING

1. **Weight-Based Dosing**
   Most pediatric medications are calculated in **mg/kg/dose** or **mg/kg/day**.

   Example:
   Amoxicillin 25–50 mg/kg/day divided every 12 hours.

2. **Age-Appropriate Formulations**
   Liquid suspensions, chewable tablets, or dissolvable forms are often preferred.
3. **Avoid Volume Overload**
   Especially important in neonates with limited fluid tolerance.
4. **Standardized Dosing Tools**
   Use calibrated syringes, oral dispensers, or infusion pumps—never household spoons.
5. **Check Maximum Adult Doses**
   Never exceed the adult maximum dose, even in older children.

HIGH-RISK DRUGS IN PEDIATRICS

Drug/Class	Risk/Concern	Nursing Consideration
Codeine	Respiratory depression; variable metabolism	Contraindicated in children under 12
Promethazine	Severe respiratory depression in <2 years	Not recommended in young children
Benzodiazepines	Sedation, apnea	Use with caution; monitor respiratory status
Antihistamines (1st gen)	Sedation, paradoxical excitation	Use lowest dose; monitor behavior
Gentamicin	Ototoxicity, nephrotoxicity	Monitor drug levels and renal function
Ceftriaxone (neonates)	Risk of biliary sludging, displacement of bilirubin	Avoid in neonates under 28 days
Tetracyclines	Tooth discoloration, impaired bone growth	Avoid in children under 8

SAFE MEDICATION ADMINISTRATION PRACTICES

- **Double-check all calculations**, especially for IV medications.
- **Verify with a second nurse** for high-alert drugs or off-label use.

- Use **age-appropriate language** when educating children or caregivers.
- Confirm patient identity and weight at each encounter.
- **Do not round doses excessively**—use precision syringes.
- **Observe closely for side effects**, especially in first-time or new-dose administrations.

PARENTAL/CAREGIVER EDUCATION TIPS

- Always use the **provided oral syringe or dropper**, not a kitchen spoon.
- Store medications **out of reach of children** in childproof containers.
- Clarify **scheduling instructions**, especially with antibiotics.
- Emphasize **adherence to full treatment courses**, even if symptoms improve.
- Watch for signs of allergy or overdose (e.g., rash, vomiting, unusual sleepiness).
- Encourage parents to call if unsure about a missed dose or incorrect administration.

COMMON PEDIATRIC DOSING TOOLS

Tool	Use
Oral syringe	Most accurate for liquid medications
Dosing cup	For older children capable of self-drinking
Medication spoon	For toddlers, marked in mL

Tool	Use
Infusion pump	For IV drugs and fluids (mL/hr or mcg/kg/min)

8.4 GERIATRIC MEDICATION MANAGEMENT

Older adults represent a growing proportion of the patient population and are the **largest consumers of prescription medications**. However, age-related physiological changes and **polypharmacy** significantly increase their risk for adverse drug reactions, drug interactions, and medication nonadherence.

Effective medication management in geriatric patients requires a thorough understanding of **age-related changes**, high-risk drug classes, and **nursing strategies tailored to safety, simplicity, and adherence**.

AGE-RELATED PHARMACOKINETIC CHANGES

Process	Age-Related Change	Impact on Medications
Absorption	Slowed gastric emptying, decreased GI blood flow	Minimal change in most drugs
Distribution	Increased fat, decreased lean body mass and total body water	Lipophilic drugs have prolonged half-life
Metabolism	Reduced hepatic enzyme activity and blood flow	Slower clearance of hepatically metabolized drugs

Process	Age-Related Change	Impact on Medications
Excretion	Decreased renal function (GFR, creatinine clearance)	Accumulation of renally cleared medications

POLYPHARMACY AND ITS RISKS

Polypharmacy (commonly defined as taking ≥5 medications) is a major contributor to:

- Adverse drug reactions (ADRs)
- Falls, delirium, and functional decline
- Drug-drug interactions
- Medication nonadherence

Nurses must routinely reconcile medications, identify potentially inappropriate drugs, and monitor for cumulative side effects.

HIGH-RISK DRUG CLASSES IN THE ELDERLY (BEERS CRITERIA)

Drug/Class	Risks in Older Adults	Nursing Considerations
Benzodiazepines	Sedation, falls, cognitive impairment	Avoid long-acting forms; use alternatives for sleep/anxiety
Anticholinergics	Confusion, urinary retention, constipation	Minimize use; assess for anticholinergic burden

Drug/Class	Risks in Older Adults	Nursing Considerations
NSAIDs	GI bleeding, renal impairment, hypertension	Use with caution; monitor renal function
Digoxin	Increased toxicity risk with renal decline	Use ≤0.125 mg/day unless otherwise indicated
Sliding-scale insulin	Hypoglycemia risk without improved outcomes	Prefer basal insulin regimens
Antipsychotics	Increased mortality in dementia-related psychosis	Use only when non-drug interventions fail
Opioids	Respiratory depression, constipation	Start low, go slow; monitor bowel function

COMMON MEDICATION SAFETY CONCERNS IN OLDER ADULTS

- **Reduced adherence** due to cost, complexity, vision, or cognition
- **Duplication** of therapies from multiple providers or pharmacies
- **Self-medication** with OTCs and supplements
- **Misunderstanding of instructions or improper timing**
- **Unrecognized side effects** mimicking aging (e.g., confusion, weakness)

NURSING ASSESSMENT AND INTERVENTIONS

1. **Medication Reconciliation**
    - Conduct at every transition of care.
    - Clarify indications, dosages, and durations.
2. **Monitor for Side Effects**
    - Be alert for atypical presentations: e.g., confusion instead of GI upset.
    - Assess balance, gait, orthostatic BP, and hydration.
3. **Simplify Regimens**
    - Recommend once-daily dosing when possible.
    - Use pill organizers, medication calendars, or blister packs.
4. **Involve the Care Team**
    - Work with pharmacists to deprescribe unnecessary medications.
    - Collaborate with providers on renal dose adjustments.
5. **Educate and Empower**
    - Use large-print materials and simple language.
    - Involve caregivers or family members as needed.
    - Encourage patients to report any new symptoms or concerns.

BEST PRACTICES FOR GERIATRIC MEDICATION SAFETY

- **Start low and go slow** when initiating or adjusting medications.
- Regularly assess **renal and hepatic function** to guide dosing.
- Review for **drug duplication or interactions** during each assessment.
- Refer to tools like the **Beers Criteria**, STOPP/START, or medication appropriateness indices.

9. CLINICAL NURSING PRACTICE

9.1 THE 10 GOLDEN RULES OF DRUG SAFETY

The administration of medications is one of the most critical responsibilities in nursing. Even minor errors in this process can lead to **severe patient harm**, particularly when dealing with high-risk drugs or vulnerable populations. The following **10 Golden Rules of Drug Safety** serve as a core framework for ensuring safe, effective, and ethical medication administration in all clinical settings.

These principles are not merely procedural—they reflect a **culture of accountability, clinical judgment, and patient advocacy.**

1. RIGHT PATIENT

- Always verify the patient's identity using **two identifiers** (e.g., full name and date of birth).
- Cross-check with the **medication administration record (MAR)** and the patient's ID band.
- Avoid assumptions, especially in shared rooms or with confused patients.

2. RIGHT DRUG

- Confirm the **generic and brand name** against the physician's order.
- Be cautious with **look-alike/sound-alike medications** (LASA).
- If unsure about the drug, **do not administer** until clarification is obtained.

3. RIGHT DOSE

- Review the order and **perform all calculations accurately**.
- Consider patient-specific factors like **age, weight, renal/hepatic function**.
- For high-alert drugs (e.g., insulin, heparin), obtain an **independent double-check**.

4. RIGHT ROUTE

- Confirm the prescribed **route of administration** (oral, IV, IM, SubQ, etc.).
- Assess whether the route is appropriate (e.g., can the patient swallow? Is the IV site patent?).
- Avoid substitutions (e.g., crushing a tablet that should not be altered) without prescriber approval.

5. RIGHT TIME

- Administer medications at the **correct time interval**, accounting for time-critical meds (e.g., antibiotics, insulin).
- Consider timing in relation to **meals, sleep, or lab draws**.
- Document exact administration times accurately.

6. RIGHT DOCUMENTATION

- Chart medications **immediately after administration**, never before.

- Include **time, dose, route, site**, and any relevant observations or patient responses.
- If a dose is withheld or refused, document **why** and notify the provider if required.

7. RIGHT REASON

- Understand the **therapeutic purpose** of each medication.
- Assess whether it is appropriate based on the patient's current condition.
- Do not administer a drug simply because it is ordered—**use clinical judgment**.

8. RIGHT RESPONSE

- Monitor for **effectiveness** (e.g., pain relief, lowered BP) and **side effects**.
- Document therapeutic outcomes and reassess as needed.
- Report any **adverse or unexpected reactions** immediately.

9. RIGHT EDUCATION

- Inform the patient about the **medication name, purpose, expected effects, and possible side effects**.
- Encourage questions and clarify misunderstandings.
- Provide **written instructions** for at-home medications when appropriate.

10. RIGHT TO REFUSE

- Recognize and respect the **patient's autonomy** to refuse any medication.
- Explore reasons for refusal in a nonjudgmental way.
- Document the refusal and notify the healthcare provider if appropriate.

ADDITIONAL SAFETY TIPS

- Avoid multitasking during med preparation—**focus reduces error**.
- Use **barcoding systems** and **smart pumps** where available.
- Report **near misses and errors** as part of a just culture focused on learning, not punishment.
- Stay current on **formulary changes, alerts, and high-alert medication updates**.

9.2 TEACHING PATIENTS ABOUT THEIR MEDICATIONS

Patient education is a fundamental part of safe and effective medication therapy. When patients understand the **purpose, timing, administration, and potential effects** of their medications, they are more likely to adhere to treatment plans, recognize side effects early, and avoid preventable complications.

Nurses are at the forefront of this process, providing accessible, personalized, and evidence-based information at the bedside, in clinics, and during discharge planning.

GOALS OF MEDICATION EDUCATION

- **Promote adherence** by ensuring patients understand why and how to take each drug.
- **Reduce medication errors** by clarifying routes, timing, and dosages.
- **Support self-management**, especially for chronic conditions.
- **Empower patients** to report adverse effects and interactions.

CORE TOPICS TO COVER WITH EACH MEDICATION

Topic	Details to Include
Medication name	Brand and generic name, pronunciation tips if needed
Purpose	Why the patient is taking it (condition or symptom targeted)
Dosage and schedule	Amount to take, frequency, with or without food, duration
Route of administration	Oral, injection, inhalation, topical, etc.
How to take it properly	Swallow whole, dissolve, shake suspension, refrigerate if needed
Common side effects	What's expected vs. when to call the provider

Topic	Details to Include
Serious adverse effects	Signs of allergic reaction, bleeding, infection, etc.
Interactions	Foods, beverages, supplements, or other drugs to avoid
Missed dose instructions	What to do and what not to do
Storage	Room temperature, refrigeration, light protection

TEACHING STRATEGIES FOR NURSES

1. INDIVIDUALIZE THE APPROACH

- Consider literacy level, language, cultural background, and learning style.
- Use **"teach-back" method** to confirm understanding:

    "Can you tell me in your own words how you'll take this at home?"

2. USE SIMPLE, CLEAR LANGUAGE

- Avoid medical jargon.
- Use plain language and short sentences.

3. SUPPLEMENT VERBAL INSTRUCTION WITH WRITTEN MATERIALS

- Provide easy-to-read medication handouts (preferably 5th–6th grade reading level).
- Highlight key points: dose, timing, major warnings.

4. REINFORCE INFORMATION OVER TIME

- Re-teach at different stages: admission, during care, and at discharge.
- Confirm understanding before initiating new medications.

5. INCLUDE CAREGIVERS WHEN NEEDED

- Involve family members or caregivers in teaching, especially for elderly, pediatric, or cognitively impaired patients.

HIGH-RISK EDUCATION SCENARIOS

- **Newly prescribed high-alert medications** (e.g., insulin, anticoagulants)
- **Medications with complex administration** (e.g., inhalers, injectables, eye drops)
- **Changes to a long-standing regimen** (e.g., dose change, brand switch)
- **Post-discharge instructions**, particularly after hospitalization or surgery

COMMON PATIENT QUESTIONS TO ANTICIPATE

- "Is it safe to take this with my other medications?"
- "What happens if I miss a dose?"
- "How will I know if this is working?"
- "Will it make me drowsy or keep me awake?"
- "Can I drink alcohol or drive while taking this?"

Provide honest, non-alarming, evidence-based answers.

DOCUMENTATION ESSENTIALS

- Document the **content and method** of education (verbal, written, demonstration).
- Record the **patient's understanding** and questions.
- Note any **refusal of instruction** or follow-up needs.

9.3 PROPER MEDICATION DOCUMENTATION

Accurate and timely documentation of medication administration is a legal, professional, and ethical obligation in nursing. It ensures **continuity of care**, supports **medication safety**, and serves as a critical record in the event of adverse events, audits, or legal review.

This section outlines the principles, standards, and best practices for proper medication documentation across different care settings.

WHY DOCUMENTATION MATTERS

- Provides a **real-time record** of what was given, when, how, and by whom.
- Enables healthcare providers to **track effectiveness and side effects**.

- Reduces **medication errors**, duplication, or missed doses.
- Serves as a **legal record** of nursing care and professional accountability.

ESSENTIAL ELEMENTS OF MEDICATION DOCUMENTATION

Component	What to Record
Drug name	Generic name preferred; brand name if specified
Dosage	Exact amount given (e.g., 5 mg, 1 mL)
Route	Oral, IV, IM, SubQ, inhaled, topical, etc.
Time and date	Exact time medication was administered
Site (if applicable)	For injections or topical meds (e.g., left deltoid, right abdomen)
Nurse's initials or ID	Verifies who administered the drug
Patient response	Especially for PRN, high-alert, or first-time medications
Omissions or delays	Reason why dose was held or not given (e.g., NPO, patient refused, low BP)
Adverse	Observed effects and any interventions taken

| Component | What to Record |

reactions

DOCUMENTATION TOOLS AND SYSTEMS

- **MAR (Medication Administration Record):**
    - May be paper or electronic (eMAR)
    - Includes scheduled, PRN, and as-needed medications
- **Barcoded systems**: Link patient ID and drug label to ensure match
- **Smart pumps and infusion records**: Capture continuous or titrated drug delivery
- **Narrative nursing notes**: Used for documenting patient response, education, or irregularities

BEST PRACTICES FOR NURSES

1. DOCUMENT IMMEDIATELY AFTER ADMINISTRATION

- Never chart in advance.
- Prevents omission, duplication, or confusion.

2. USE APPROVED ABBREVIATIONS ONLY

- Avoid dangerous shorthand (e.g., "U" for units, "QD" for daily).
- Refer to your institution's list of approved terms.

3. BE ACCURATE AND OBJECTIVE

- Use precise language. Avoid subjective phrases like "patient seemed fine"—describe what you observed.
- Example: "Patient reports pain relief 20 minutes post-IV morphine 2 mg."

4. CHART REFUSALS AND MISSED DOSES

- Include the reason (e.g., "patient refused due to nausea") and your follow-up actions.
- Notify provider when necessary and document the communication.

5. RECORD PRN MEDICATIONS CLEARLY

- Include the **indication, time given**, and **patient's response**.
- Example: "Acetaminophen 650 mg PO at 1400 for fever of 38.5°C; temp reduced to 37.8°C at 1500."

6. DOCUMENT ADVERSE REACTIONS PROMPTLY

- Include symptoms, interventions, and provider notification.
- Document monitoring post-reaction.

COMMON DOCUMENTATION PITFALLS TO AVOID

- **Omitting time or route** of administration
- **Failing to record patient response** to PRN or high-alert medications
- **Illegible handwriting** (in paper records)
- **Using unapproved abbreviations**
- **Pre-charting** doses not yet given

LEGAL AND ETHICAL CONSIDERATIONS

- Your documentation may be reviewed in **legal cases, audits, or regulatory investigations**.
- If it's **not documented, it's considered not done**.
- Altering records or failing to document accurately can result in **disciplinary action or litigation**.

10. DOSAGE & IV CALCULATIONS CHEAT SHEET

10.1 WEIGHT-BASED & PEDIATRIC DOSING

In many clinical scenarios—particularly in **pediatrics, oncology, critical care, and obesity management**—medication dosages must be calculated based on the patient's **body weight or body surface area (BSA)**. This ensures that the dosage is **therapeutically effective yet safe**, avoiding toxicity or underdosing.

This section provides a practical reference for calculating weight-based doses, including formulas, common conversions, and key nursing considerations for safe administration.

WHY WEIGHT-BASED DOSING MATTERS

- Pediatric patients have immature organ systems that affect drug metabolism and excretion.
- Some medications (e.g., **aminoglycosides, insulin, chemotherapy agents**) have **narrow therapeutic windows**.

- Obese or underweight patients require tailored dosing based on **actual body weight (ABW), ideal body weight (IBW), or adjusted body weight (AdjBW).**

STANDARD WEIGHT-BASED DOSING FORMULA

$$\text{Dose (mg)} = \text{mg/kg} \times \text{Weight (kg)}$$

- Always **convert weight from pounds to kilograms** when needed:

$$kg = \frac{lb}{2.2}$$

EXAMPLE CALCULATION

Order: Cefazolin 25 mg/kg IV every 8 hours
Patient weight: 22 lb

1. Convert weight:
   22 ÷ 2.2 = **10 kg**
2. Calculate dose:
   25 mg × 10 kg = **250 mg per dose**

BODY SURFACE AREA (BSA) DOSING FORMULA

Used especially in **chemotherapy and high-risk drugs**:

$$\text{BSA (m}^2\text{)} = \sqrt{\frac{\text{Height (cm)} \times \text{Weight (kg)}}{3600}}$$

$$\text{Dose (mg)} = \text{mg/m}^2 \times \text{BSA}$$

USE BSA CALCULATORS OR DRUG-SPECIFIC PROTOCOLS FOR ACCURACY.

IDEAL BODY WEIGHT (IBW) FORMULA

Used in adult dosing for certain medications (e.g., aminoglycosides):

- **Male:**

    $$\text{IBW} = 50 + 2.3 \times (\text{height in inches} - 60)$$

- **Female:**

    $$\text{IBW} = 45.5 + 2.3 \times (\text{height in inches} - 60)$$

ADJUSTED BODY WEIGHT (ADJBW)

Used when actual body weight is significantly higher than IBW:

$$\text{AdjBW} = \text{IBW} + 0.4 \times (\text{ABW} - \text{IBW})$$

COMMON PEDIATRIC DOSING GUIDELINES (SELECTED EXAMPLES)

Medication	Dose Range	Route	Note
Acetaminophen	10–15 mg/kg every 4–6 hrs	PO/PR	Max 75 mg/kg/day
Ibuprofen	5–10 mg/kg every 6–8 hrs	PO	Use in children >6 months
Amoxicillin	25–50 mg/kg/day in divided doses	PO	Adjust based on infection severity
Gentamicin	2.5 mg/kg every 8 hrs	IV	Monitor peaks/troughs and renal function
Epinephrine (anaphylaxis)	0.01 mg/kg IM (max 0.3 mg)	IM	Use 1:1,000 concentration

NURSING CONSIDERATIONS

- **Double-check all calculations**, especially for pediatrics and high-alert meds.
- Use **standard dosing references** (e.g., Harriet Lane, Lexicomp Pediatric, institutional protocols).
- Always **confirm units** (mg vs mcg) and **volume equivalents**.
- Document **dose rationale** and response clearly in the chart.
- For IV meds, assess if dosing is per **dose or per day** and divide accordingly.

- **Round cautiously**—do not round up beyond safe limits for neonates and infants.

10.2 IV FLOW RATE CALCULATIONS

Accurate intravenous (IV) flow rate calculation is essential to ensure that medications and fluids are delivered at the **correct speed and volume**. Improper infusion rates can result in **underdosing, toxicity, fluid overload, or cardiovascular compromise**—especially in critical care, pediatric, and geriatric populations.

This section provides formulas and clinical examples to help nurses confidently calculate **manual (gravity) and pump-based** IV infusion rates.

I. IV FLOW RATE (ML/HR) – FOR IV PUMPS

Used when administering fluids or medications via an infusion pump.

Formula:

$$\text{Flow rate (mL/hr)} = \frac{\text{Total volume (mL)}}{\text{Time (hr)}}$$

EXAMPLE:

Infuse 1,000 mL over 8 hours.

$$\frac{1{,}000 \ \text{mL}}{8 \ \text{hr}} = 125 \ \text{mL/hr}$$

II. IV DRIP RATE (GTT/MIN) – FOR MANUAL GRAVITY DRIPS

Used when controlling the infusion rate manually with a roller clamp.

Formula:

$$\text{Drip rate (gtt/min)} = \frac{\text{Total volume (mL)} \times \text{Drop factor (gtt/mL)}}{\text{Time (min)}}$$

DROP FACTOR IS BASED ON IV TUBING SET (E.G., 10, 15, 20, OR 60 GTT/ML)

EXAMPLE:

Infuse 500 mL over 4 hours using tubing with a drop factor of 20 gtt/mL.

Convert 4 hours to minutes:
4 × 60 = 240 minutes

$$\frac{500 \times 20}{240} = \frac{10{,}000}{240} = 41.6 \approx 42 \text{ gtt/min}$$

III. CALCULATING INFUSION TIME

Formula:

$$\text{Infusion time (hr)} = \frac{\text{Total volume (mL)}}{\text{Rate (mL/hr)}}$$

EXAMPLE:

Infusing 750 mL at 100 mL/hr:

$$\frac{750}{100} = 7.5 \text{ hr} = 7 \text{ hours and 30 minutes}$$

IV. WEIGHT-BASED INFUSIONS (MCG/KG/MIN OR MG/KG/HR)

Common in **critical care**, such as for vasopressors, insulin, or heparin.

Formula (basic):

$$\text{Rate (mL/hr)} = \frac{\text{Dose (mcg/kg/min)} \times \text{Weight (kg)} \times 60}{\text{Concentration (mcg/mL)}}$$

EXAMPLE:

Dopamine ordered at 5 mcg/kg/min
Patient weighs 70 kg
Bag concentration: 400 mg in 250 mL = 1,600 mcg/mL

$$\text{Rate} = \frac{5 \times 70 \times 60}{1,600} = \frac{21,000}{1,600} = 13.1 \text{ mL/hr}$$

V. TITRATING IV DRIPS (NURSING CONSIDERATIONS)

- Always use **smart pumps** for high-risk drugs (e.g., insulin, heparin, vasoactive agents).
- **Double-check calculations** for dose and rate before adjusting.

- Follow **titration protocols**: adjust incrementally, monitor vitals and labs (e.g., glucose for insulin, aPTT for heparin).
- Document each **rate change, response, and time**.

COMMON DROP FACTORS (IV TUBING SETS)

Set Type	Drop Factor (gtt/mL)
Macrodrip	10, 15, or 20
Microdrip (Pediatric/Precision)**	60

ALWAYS VERIFY THE DROP FACTOR PRINTED ON THE IV TUBING PACKAGE.

QUICK REFERENCE TABLE

Volume	Time	Pump Rate (mL/hr)
1,000 mL	8 hr	125 mL/hr
500 mL	4 hr	125 mL/hr
1,000 mL	12 hr	83 mL/hr
1,000 mL	24 hr	42 mL/hr

10.3 COMMON CONVERSION CHARTS

Safe medication administration often requires converting between **units of measurement**. Whether adjusting for weight, volume, time, or dosage units, nurses must be fluent in these conversions to prevent calculation errors that could lead to underdosing or overdosing.

This section provides a concise, easy-to-reference set of **conversion tables and formulas** used daily in nursing practice.

A. WEIGHT CONVERSIONS

To Convert	Multiply by	Equals
Pounds (lb) → Kilograms (kg)	0.45	1 lb = 0.45 kg
Kilograms (kg) → Pounds (lb)	2.2	1 kg = 2.2 lb
Grams (g) → Milligrams (mg)	1,000	1 g = 1,000 mg
Milligrams (mg) → Micrograms (mcg)	1,000	1 mg = 1,000 mcg
Micrograms (mcg) → Milligrams (mg)	0.001	1 mcg = 0.001 mg

B. VOLUME CONVERSIONS

To Convert	Multiply by	Equals
Liters (L) → Milliliters (mL)	1,000	1 L = 1,000 mL
Milliliters (mL) → Liters (L)	0.001	1 mL = 0.001 L
Teaspoon (tsp) → Milliliters	5	1 tsp = 5 mL
Tablespoon (tbsp) → Milliliters	15	1 tbsp = 15 mL
Ounce (oz) → Milliliters	30	1 oz = 30 mL
Cup (U.S.) → Milliliters	240	1 cup = 240 mL

C. TIME CONVERSIONS

To Convert	Equals
1 hour	60 minutes
1 day	24 hours
1 week	7 days

To Convert	Equals
1 month (approx.)	30 days

D. TEMPERATURE CONVERSIONS

Formula	Use Case
°F to °C: (°F − 32) × 5 ÷ 9 = °C	Converting body temp to Celsius
°C to °F: (°C × 9 ÷ 5) + 32 = °F	Converting Celsius to Fahrenheit

E. UNITS OF MEASURE IN DRUG DOSING

Unit	Definition
mEq	Milliequivalents; used for electrolytes like K^+, Na^+
IU	International Units; used for vitamins, insulin
Units	Measurement of biological activity (e.g., insulin, heparin)
% Solution	g/100 mL (e.g., 5% dextrose = 5 g dextrose per 100 mL)

Unit	Definition
Ratio	g/mL (e.g., 1:1,000 = 1 g in 1,000 mL)

F. COMMON ABBREVIATIONS FOR CONVERSIONS

Abbreviation	Meaning
mg	milligram
mcg	microgram
g	gram
mL	milliliter
L	liter
tsp	teaspoon
tbsp	tablespoon
oz	ounce
qd	once daily

Abbreviation	Meaning
bid	twice daily
tid	three times daily
qid	four times daily

NURSING TIPS FOR SAFE CONVERSIONS

- Always double-check unit conversions for **high-alert medications**.
- Do not confuse **mg** with **mcg**—a common and dangerous error.
- Use **leading zeros** (e.g., 0.5 mg), and avoid **trailing zeros** (e.g., 5.0 mg).
- When converting between systems (e.g., household to metric), always round **to safe dosing levels**.
- Use **institution-approved calculators** or conversion tools for accuracy.

11. CLINICAL CASE STUDIES

11.1 REAL-WORLD MEDICATION ERRORS

Despite advances in safety systems, **medication errors remain one of the most common preventable causes of patient harm** in healthcare. These errors can occur at any stage—prescribing, transcribing, dispensing, administering, or monitoring—and often result from system failures, distractions, or human error.

This section presents real-world case examples that illustrate how and why errors happen, followed by **nursing-focused lessons and prevention strategies**.

CASE STUDY 1: WRONG DOSE – HEPARIN OVERDOSE IN NEONATE

Scenario:
A neonatal ICU nurse administered **1,000 units/mL** heparin instead of the intended **10 units/mL flush** for a central line in a premature infant. The pharmacy had stocked both concentrations in similar vials.

Outcome:
The infant experienced severe bleeding and required transfusions and extended hospitalization.

Root Causes:

- Look-alike vials (LASA error)
- Inadequate labeling and segregation of high-alert meds

Nursing Takeaways:

- Always **verify concentrations**, especially with high-alert meds.
- Follow **facility protocols for independent double-checks**.
- Advocate for **barcode scanning** and **segregated storage** of similar products.

CASE STUDY 2: WRONG PATIENT – OPIOID GIVEN TO ROOMMATE

Scenario:
A nurse administered oxycodone to the wrong patient after entering a semi-private room and assuming the person sitting up was the correct recipient.

Outcome:
The unintended patient experienced oversedation requiring naloxone.

Root Causes:

- Failure to verify patient ID
- Distraction and assumption

Nursing Takeaways:

- Use **two patient identifiers** before every administration—every time.
- Never rely on **bed placement or appearance**.
- Educate float staff or new team members on **unit routines and patient layouts**.

CASE STUDY 3: MISSED DRUG INTERACTION – BLEEDING WITH WARFARIN & GINKGO

Scenario:
A patient on warfarin was admitted after experiencing a GI bleed. Upon review, it was discovered they had recently started taking **ginkgo biloba** for memory support—information that was not collected during admission.

Outcome:
The patient required transfusions and ICU monitoring.

Root Causes:

- Incomplete medication history
- Lack of supplement screening

Nursing Takeaways:

- Ask specifically about **herbal and OTC supplements**.
- Include caregivers in medication interviews if patients are forgetful.
- Educate patients about **natural product interactions** with anticoagulants.

CASE STUDY 4: WRONG ROUTE – ORAL MED CRUSHED AND GIVEN VIA NG TUBE

Scenario:
A nurse crushed an extended-release (XR) medication and administered it via a nasogastric (NG) tube, unaware that crushing the tablet would compromise its slow-release mechanism.

Outcome:
The patient experienced dose dumping, severe hypotension, and required ICU care.

Root Causes:

- Lack of awareness of dosage form
- No consultation with pharmacy

Nursing Takeaways:

- Always verify if medications can be **crushed, split, or administered via tube**.
- Use institutional **crushability lists or drug reference guides**.

- Involve the **pharmacist** when in doubt.

CASE STUDY 5: DOSE CALCULATION ERROR – PEDIATRIC VANCOMYCIN OVERDOSE

Scenario:
A 6-year-old child received a vancomycin dose based on the **adult dose of 1 gram** rather than the weight-based pediatric dose.

Outcome:
The child developed nephrotoxicity requiring renal monitoring and temporary dialysis.

Root Causes:

- Use of adult dosing without weight adjustment
- Lack of pediatric drug reference

Nursing Takeaways:

- Always use **mg/kg calculations** for pediatric patients.
- Refer to **pediatric-specific drug guides** (e.g., Lexicomp Pediatric, Harriet Lane).
- Verify doses with pharmacists for high-risk drugs in children.

COMMON THEMES IN MEDICATION ERRORS

- **Assumptions** replacing verification
- **Poor communication** or handoffs
- **Distractions** and multitasking during preparation
- Incomplete **medication history**

- **Documentation lapses** or time pressures

NURSING STRATEGIES TO PREVENT ERRORS

- Use the **"10 Rights"** of medication administration
- Slow down and **focus fully during med prep**
- Always verify **dose, route, and patient identity**
- Participate in **safety huddles, training, and simulation drills**
- Encourage **near-miss reporting** to prevent future harm

11.2 MANAGING REACTIONS IN PRACTICE

Adverse drug reactions (ADRs) can occur with any medication, at any time, and in any patient. While some are mild and self-limited, others can be severe or life-threatening. Nurses are often the first to recognize these events and are responsible for initiating timely interventions to **reduce harm and stabilize the patient.**

This section provides a step-by-step clinical guide for recognizing, assessing, managing, and documenting medication reactions across care settings.

STEP 1: RECOGNIZE THE REACTION

Be alert to **early signs and symptoms** of common ADRs:

System Affected	Warning Signs
Skin	Rash, itching, flushing, urticaria

System Affected	Warning Signs
Respiratory	Wheezing, stridor, dyspnea, throat tightness
Cardiovascular	Hypotension, tachycardia, syncope
Gastrointestinal	Nausea, vomiting, diarrhea, abdominal pain
Neurologic	Dizziness, confusion, agitation, seizures
General	Fever, chills, anaphylaxis symptoms

☐ **Tip**: If the reaction occurs soon after administration—**assume the drug is the cause** until proven otherwise.

STEP 2: STOP THE OFFENDING MEDICATION

- **Immediately discontinue** the suspected medication if a reaction is identified.
- Maintain IV access (do not remove unless extravasation is suspected).
- Do **not restart the medication** unless cleared by the prescriber.

STEP 3: ASSESS AND STABILIZE THE PATIENT

- Perform a **rapid assessment**: airway, breathing, circulation (ABCs).
- Check **vital signs** and perform a focused physical exam.

- Identify **severity**:
    - o **Mild**: localized rash, nausea
    - o **Moderate**: hypotension, bronchospasm
    - o **Severe**: anaphylaxis, respiratory arrest, seizures

STEP 4: NOTIFY THE PROVIDER AND COLLABORATE

- Report all findings, including:
    - o Medication name, dose, route, time
    - o Description of reaction and onset
    - o Vital signs and any treatments provided
- Follow any new orders (e.g., antihistamines, steroids, fluids, transfer to ICU).
- Consider activating **Rapid Response Team** if symptoms worsen.

STEP 5: ADMINISTER EMERGENCY MEDICATIONS (IF ORDERED)

Medication	Indication	Nursing Notes
Epinephrine IM	Anaphylaxis	0.3–0.5 mg IM (adults); repeat every 5–15 min
Diphenhydramine IV/PO	Urticaria, itching	Monitor sedation, BP
Methylprednisolone IV	Inflammation, airway swelling	Delayed effect; often part of sustained management

Medication	Indication	Nursing Notes
Albuterol (neb)	Bronchospasm	Monitor breath sounds, O_2 sat
IV fluids	Hypotension	Start with NS or LR; monitor for fluid overload
Oxygen	Respiratory distress	Titrate to maintain sat > 94%

STEP 6: DOCUMENT THOROUGHLY AND ACCURATELY

- Describe:
    - Onset, timing, and appearance of symptoms
    - Interventions and response
    - Communication with provider
- Update:
    - **MAR and allergy lists**
    - Patient's chart and handoff reports

☐ **Include whether this was a known allergy or a new adverse event.**

STEP 7: EDUCATE THE PATIENT AND FAMILY

- Explain what happened in **clear, non-alarming terms**.
- Advise what symptoms to report in the future.
- Stress the importance of **informing all providers** of the reaction.
- Provide or request a **medic alert bracelet** or documentation for discharge.

STEP 8: REPORT THE EVENT

- Submit an **internal incident report** per facility policy.
- Report serious ADRs to:
    - **FDA MedWatch**: www.fda.gov/medwatch
    - **ISMP** for medication safety concerns

CLINICAL TIPS FOR PREVENTION

- Always ask about **allergies and previous reactions**—including herbal products.
- Monitor closely after giving:
    - **First-time doses**
    - **IV antibiotics**
    - **High-alert meds (opioids, chemo, insulin)**
- Use **pre-medications** when ordered (e.g., before blood transfusion or contrast dye).

11.3 MEDICATION SAFETY IN ACTION

Medication safety is not just a theory—it's a daily practice that nurses implement at the bedside, during rounds, and across the continuum of care. This section highlights how nurses apply **critical thinking, protocols, and evidence-based strategies** to prevent harm and ensure medication therapy is safe and effective in real clinical situations.

CASE-BASED APPLICATIONS OF MEDICATION SAFETY

A. PREVENTING A WRONG-TIME ANTIBIOTIC ERROR

Scenario: A nurse notices that a preoperative dose of cefazolin is scheduled an hour too early for optimal surgical prophylaxis.

Nursing Action:

- Cross-checks protocol, recognizes timing discrepancy.
- Clarifies with provider and adjusts the administration time to 30 minutes pre-incision.

Impact:
Reduces risk of postoperative infection, complies with evidence-based practice.

B. INTERCEPTING A POTENTIAL OVERDOSE

Scenario: A patient with impaired renal function is prescribed a standard dose of vancomycin. The nurse reviews recent labs and finds elevated creatinine.

Nursing Action:

- Holds administration and contacts provider.
- Collaborates with pharmacy to adjust dose based on renal function.

Impact:
Prevents nephrotoxicity and supports safe individualized therapy.

C. IMPROVING SAFETY THROUGH EDUCATION

Scenario: A patient with low health literacy is being discharged with a complex insulin regimen.

Nursing Action:

- Uses visual aids and simple language to explain dosing.
- Demonstrates injection technique and uses teach-back to confirm understanding.

Impact:
Reduces risk of hypoglycemia and promotes medication adherence.

D. ADDRESSING A SYSTEM-LEVEL HAZARD

Scenario: A nurse notes that look-alike vials of potassium chloride and normal saline are stored side-by-side in the medication room.

Nursing Action:

- Reports the concern through the unit's safety system.
- Participates in a safety committee meeting that leads to improved storage practices and labeling.

Impact:
System-wide risk mitigation that protects all patients on the unit.

EVERYDAY NURSING ACTIONS THAT PROMOTE MEDICATION SAFETY

Action	Safety Contribution
Double-checking high-alert meds	Catches errors before they reach the patient
Clarifying unclear orders	Prevents misinterpretation and wrong drug administration
Scanning barcodes correctly	Ensures 5 rights are verified electronically
Reviewing allergies and interactions	Avoids preventable reactions
Educating patients on their meds	Promotes adherence and early recognition of side effects
Monitoring vitals before/after meds	Detects adverse effects early
Accurately documenting doses and responses	Provides legal protection and continuity of care

USING TECHNOLOGY FOR SAFETY

- **Smart infusion pumps**: Reduce IV rate errors with built-in drug libraries.

- **Electronic Medication Administration Records (eMAR)**: Prevent missed or duplicate doses.
- **Clinical decision support systems**: Flag allergies, interactions, and dosage outliers.

HOWEVER, TECHNOLOGY NEVER REPLACES CRITICAL THINKING—NURSES MUST ALWAYS ASSESS, VERIFY, AND ADVOCATE.

FOSTERING A CULTURE OF SAFETY

- Report **near misses** and actual errors without fear of punishment.
- Encourage **open communication** among the care team.
- Participate in **medication safety rounds**, committees, or quality improvement projects.
- Stay **current with guidelines**, black box warnings, and formulary updates.

12. APPENDICES & RESOURCES

12.1 COMMON ABBREVIATIONS IN PHARMACOLOGY

Pharmacological documentation often includes abbreviations that **streamline communication** across healthcare settings. While standardized abbreviations improve efficiency, improper use or misinterpretation can lead to **serious medication errors**.

This appendix provides a reference list of **approved and commonly used pharmacology abbreviations** nurses may encounter in practice. It also highlights **dangerous abbreviations** that should be avoided, as recommended by the **Joint Commission and ISMP (Institute for Safe Medication Practices)**.

A. GENERAL ABBREVIATIONS

Abbreviation	Meaning
Rx	Prescription
Dx	Diagnosis
Tx	Treatment
Hx	History
Sx	Symptoms

Abbreviation	Meaning
PRN	As needed
Stat	Immediately
NPO	Nothing by mouth
PO	By mouth (oral)
IV	Intravenous
IM	Intramuscular
SubQ	Subcutaneous
SL	Sublingual
gtt	Drops
q	Every
qd	Every day
bid	Twice daily

Abbreviation	Meaning
tid	Three times daily
qid	Four times daily
ac	Before meals
pc	After meals
hs	At bedtime
AU, AD, AS	Both ears, right ear, left ear
OU, OD, OS	Both eyes, right eye, left eye

B. UNITS OF MEASUREMENT

Abbreviation	Meaning
mg	Milligram
g	Gram
mcg	Microgram

Abbreviation	Meaning
mEq	Milliequivalent
mL	Milliliter
L	Liter
IU	International Unit
kg	Kilogram
lb	Pound

C. DRUG ADMINISTRATION TIMING

Abbreviation	Meaning
q4h	Every 4 hours
q6h	Every 6 hours
q8h	Every 8 hours
q12h	Every 12 hours

Abbreviation	Meaning
qd	Once daily (use with caution)
qod	Every other day (discouraged)
qwk	Every week
qhs	Every night at bedtime
prn	As needed

D. ROUTES OF ADMINISTRATION

Abbreviation	Route
PO	Oral
IM	Intramuscular
IV	Intravenous
ID	Intradermal
SubQ	Subcutaneous

Abbreviation	Route
PR	Per rectum
SL	Sublingual
Top	Topical
INH	Inhalation
NG	Nasogastric

E. DANGEROUS ABBREVIATIONS TO AVOID

Avoid	Use Instead	Why?
U	Unit	Can be mistaken for "0" or "4"
IU	International Unit	Mistaken for IV or 10
QD, QOD	Daily, Every other day	Mistaken for each other
.5 mg	0.5 mg	Decimal point may be missed
5.0 mg	5 mg	Trailing zero may be misread as 50 mg

Avoid	Use Instead	Why?
MS, MSO4	Morphine sulfate	Can be confused with magnesium sulfate
MgSO4	Magnesium sulfate	May be mistaken for morphine sulfate

☐ **Note**: Always follow your facility's approved abbreviation list and avoid unapproved shorthand in documentation and orders.

F. COMMON LATIN ROOTS STILL IN USE

Abbreviation	Latin	Meaning
ac	ante cibum	Before meals
pc	post cibum	After meals
hs	hora somni	At bedtime
prn	pro re nata	As needed
q	quaque	Every
bid	bis in die	Twice a day
tid	ter in die	Three times a day

Abbreviation	Latin	Meaning
qid	quater in die	Four times a day

12.2 GLOSSARY OF KEY TERMS

This glossary provides definitions of **core pharmacological and nursing terms** commonly used throughout clinical practice. It serves as a quick reference to support **clarity, consistency, and safe medication administration** in all healthcare settings.

A

- **Absorption** – The process by which a drug enters the bloodstream from the site of administration.
- **Adverse Drug Reaction (ADR)** – An unintended and harmful response to a medication at normal doses.
- **Agonist** – A drug that binds to a receptor and activates it to produce a biological response.
- **Antagonist** – A drug that blocks or inhibits the action of an agonist at a receptor site.
- **Anaphylaxis** – A severe, life-threatening allergic reaction requiring immediate intervention.

B

- **Bioavailability** – The percentage of a drug dose that reaches systemic circulation and is available for action.
- **Black Box Warning** – The strictest warning by the FDA, indicating serious or life-threatening drug risks.
- **Bolus** – A single, often rapid, dose of medication administered intravenously.

C

- **Contraindication** – A specific situation in which a drug should not be used due to risk of harm.
- **Cumulative Effect** – An increased effect of a drug when doses are given in succession before the body can eliminate prior doses.

D

- **Drug Interaction** – A modification in drug effect due to the presence of another drug, food, or substance.
- **Drug Half-Life (t½)** – The time required for half of a drug to be eliminated from the body.

E

- **Enteral Route** – Administration of drugs via the gastrointestinal tract (oral, sublingual, rectal).
- **Excretion** – The process of eliminating drugs from the body, primarily via the kidneys.

F

- **First-Pass Effect** – The metabolism of a drug in the liver before it reaches systemic circulation when taken orally.
- **Formulary** – A list of approved medications maintained by a healthcare institution or insurance plan.

H

- **High-Alert Medication** – A drug that carries a higher risk of causing significant harm if used incorrectly.
- **Hypersensitivity Reaction** – An exaggerated immune response to a drug, which can range from mild to severe.

I

- **Idiosyncratic Reaction** – An abnormal or unexpected drug response, often due to genetic variation.
- **Infusion** – Continuous delivery of fluids or medication over a period of time via intravenous access.

L

- **Loading Dose** – A higher initial dose of a drug used to rapidly achieve therapeutic levels.

M

- **Maintenance Dose** – A regular dose given to maintain the desired drug concentration.
- **Medication Reconciliation** – The process of ensuring medication accuracy across transitions in care.
- **Metabolism** – The body's process of chemically converting a drug into an active or inactive form.

O

- **Onset of Action** – The time it takes for a drug to produce a therapeutic effect after administration.

P

- **Parenteral Route** – Non-oral routes of drug administration, typically injectable (e.g., IV, IM, SubQ).
- **Peak Level** – The highest concentration of a drug in the bloodstream after administration.
- **Pharmacodynamics** – The study of what a drug does to the body (mechanism of action).
- **Pharmacokinetics** – The study of what the body does to a drug (absorption, distribution, metabolism, excretion).
- **Placebo** – An inactive substance used in clinical trials to compare against an active drug.

S

- **Side Effect** – An expected but non-therapeutic response to a drug; may be beneficial, neutral, or harmful.

- **Steady State** – The point at which the drug intake equals drug elimination, maintaining consistent blood levels.
- **Synergistic Effect** – When two drugs combined have a greater effect than either alone.

T

- **Therapeutic Range** – The range of drug concentration in the blood that provides effectiveness without toxicity.
- **Tolerance** – A reduced response to a drug over time, requiring higher doses for the same effect.
- **Toxicity** – Harmful effects of a drug resulting from excessive dosage or prolonged use.
- **Trough Level** – The lowest concentration of a drug in the bloodstream, usually measured just before the next dose.

V

- **Vesicant** – A drug that can cause tissue damage if it leaks into surrounding tissue (extravasation).
- **Volume of Distribution (Vd)** – A pharmacokinetic parameter describing the extent to which a drug spreads in the body.

12.3 CONVERSION CHARTS & UNITS

Accurate medication administration depends on the nurse's ability to convert between various **units of weight, volume, time, and drug concentrations**. Miscalculations can lead to incorrect dosages with serious patient consequences—especially in pediatrics, critical care, and IV therapy.

This section provides quick-reference **conversion tables** and standard units used in medication dosing and nursing practice.

A. METRIC SYSTEM CONVERSIONS

From	To	Conversion
1 gram (g)	milligrams (mg)	1 g = 1,000 mg
1 milligram (mg)	micrograms (mcg)	1 mg = 1,000 mcg
1 kilogram (kg)	grams (g)	1 kg = 1,000 g
1 liter (L)	milliliters (mL)	1 L = 1,000 mL
1 milliliter (mL)	cubic centimeters (cc)	1 mL = 1 cc

☐ TIP: ALWAYS USE METRIC UNITS WHEN PREPARING AND ADMINISTERING MEDICATIONS.

B. HOUSEHOLD TO METRIC EQUIVALENTS

Household Measure	Metric Equivalent
1 teaspoon (tsp)	5 mL

Household Measure	Metric Equivalent
1 tablespoon (tbsp)	15 mL
1 ounce (oz)	30 mL
1 cup (U.S.)	240 mL
1 pint	480 mL (approx.)
1 quart	960 mL (approx.)
1 pound (lb)	454 grams (g) or 0.45 kg

☐ Household utensils are **not reliable** for measuring medication. Always provide patients with calibrated dosing devices.

C. WEIGHT CONVERSIONS

From	To	Conversion
Pounds (lb)	Kilograms (kg)	Divide by 2.2
Kilograms (kg)	Pounds (lb)	Multiply by 2.2

D. TIME CONVERSIONS

From	To	Conversion
1 hour	60 minutes	
1 day	24 hours	
1 week	7 days	
1 month	30 days (approx.)	

E. TEMPERATURE CONVERSIONS

Formula	Use
°F → °C: (°F − 32) × 5 ÷ 9 = °C	Convert Fahrenheit to Celsius
°C → °F: (°C × 9 ÷ 5) + 32 = °F	Convert Celsius to Fahrenheit

F. IV FLUID AND FLOW RATE BASICS

Conversion	Value
1 liter (L)	1,000 milliliters (mL)

Conversion	Value
Drops per mL (macrodrip)	10, 15, or 20 gtt/mL
Drops per mL (microdrip)	60 gtt/mL
1 hour	60 minutes
IV rate (mL/hr)	Volume ÷ Time (hours)
Drip rate (gtt/min)	(mL × drop factor) ÷ time (min)

G. COMMON ABBREVIATIONS FOR UNITS

Abbreviation	Unit
g	Gram
mg	Milligram
mcg	Microgram
mEq	Milliequivalent
mL	Milliliter

Abbreviation	Unit
L	Liter
IU	International Unit
U	Unit (use with caution)

☐ Avoid using "U" for units in handwritten notes—can be mistaken for "0" (use "units" instead).

H. DOSAGE STRENGTH CONVERSION EXAMPLE

Order: Administer 250 mg of medication.
Available: 500 mg/2 mL vial.

$$\text{Volume to give} = \frac{250\ mg}{500\ mg} \times 2\ mL = 1\ mL$$

12.4 Most Commonly Prescribed Drugs (U.S. 2025)

12.4 MOST COMMONLY PRESCRIBED DRUGS (U.S. 2025)

Understanding the most frequently prescribed medications provides nurses with valuable insight into **prevailing health conditions**, **medication trends**, and **patient safety priorities**. These drugs are encountered daily across various clinical settings, from primary care to critical care.

This list includes the **top prescribed medications in the U.S. in 2025**, based on data from national pharmacy networks, insurance claim analysis, and FDA reporting. It covers each drug's **generic and brand names, primary indications, and key nursing considerations**.

TOP 25 MOST COMMONLY PRESCRIBED DRUGS IN 2025

Generic Name	Brand Name	Primary Use	Nursing Considerations
Atorvastatin	Lipitor®	Hyperlipidemia	Monitor liver enzymes; assess for myopathy
Lisinopril	Prinivil®, Zestril®	Hypertension, heart failure	Monitor BP, potassium; caution in renal impairment
Levothyroxine	Synthroid®, Levoxyl®	Hypothyroidism	Take on empty stomach; monitor TSH regularly
Metformin	Glucophage®	Type 2 diabetes	Hold if contrast dye used; monitor for GI upset and lactic

Generic Name	Brand Name	Primary Use	Nursing Considerations
			acidosis
Amlodipine	Norvasc®	Hypertension, angina	Monitor BP, edema; patient may report dizziness
Omeprazole	Prilosec®	GERD, ulcers	Take before meals; avoid long-term use without evaluation
Losartan	Cozaar®	Hypertension, kidney protection in diabetes	Monitor BP, potassium
Simvastatin	Zocor®	Hyperlipidemia	Administer in the evening; avoid grapefruit
Albuterol (inhaled)	Ventolin®, ProAir®	Asthma, COPD	Assess lung sounds pre/post; rinse mouth after use

Generic Name	Brand Name	Primary Use	Nursing Considerations
Gabapentin	Neurontin®	Neuropathy, seizures	May cause sedation; taper if discontinuing
Hydrocodone/Acetaminophen	Norco®, Vicodin®	Moderate pain	Monitor for sedation, constipation; controlled substance
Sertraline	Zoloft®	Depression, anxiety	Monitor for serotonin syndrome; assess mood regularly
Fluticasone (inhaled)	Flovent®	Asthma maintenance	Rinse mouth after use; not for acute attacks
Amoxicillin	Amoxil®	Bacterial infections	Assess for allergy; take full course
Prednisone	Deltasone®	Inflammation, autoimmune	Monitor glucose, mood, taper if long-

Generic Name	Brand Name	Primary Use	Nursing Considerations
			term use
Tamsulosin	Flomax®	BPH	Administer after meals; watch for orthostatic hypotension
Escitalopram	Lexapro®	Depression, anxiety	Onset may take weeks; monitor for suicidal ideation
Clopidogrel	Plavix®	Antiplatelet	Monitor for bleeding; avoid with NSAIDs
Insulin glargine	Lantus®, Basaglar®	Diabetes (basal insulin)	Monitor blood glucose; do not mix with other insulins
Furosemide	Lasix®	Edema, hypertension	Monitor K+, BP, daily weights; administer in morning

Generic Name	Brand Name	Primary Use	Nursing Considerations
Montelukast	Singulair®	Asthma, allergies	Take in evening; not for acute symptoms
Bupropion	Wellbutrin®	Depression, smoking cessation	Take in AM; seizure risk at high doses
Acetaminophen	Tylenol®	Mild pain, fever	Monitor total daily dose (max 4g/day); hepatotoxicity risk
Duloxetine	Cymbalta®	Depression, neuropathy	Monitor BP, mood; assess liver function
Cetirizine	Zyrtec®	Allergic rhinitis	Non-sedating; may still cause drowsiness in some patients

KEY NURSING IMPLICATIONS ACROSS HIGH-USE MEDICATIONS

- **Assess for drug-drug interactions**, especially with polypharmacy in older adults.
- Monitor for **adherence**, particularly with chronic conditions like hypertension or diabetes.
- Educate patients on **timing, side effects, and lifestyle modifications** that support medication effectiveness.
- Reinforce **black box warnings** and **patient safety alerts** (e.g., SSRIs and suicidal ideation in young adults).
- Document **patient response, teaching, and adverse effects** meticulously.

CONCLUSION

These commonly prescribed medications reflect national treatment trends for **cardiovascular disease, mental health, metabolic disorders, and respiratory conditions**. Nurses must be familiar with their indications, dosing nuances, and patient teaching priorities to ensure safe, effective care in every setting.

Made in United States
Troutdale, OR
06/19/2025